Therapeutic Games
and Guided Imagery

Therapeutic Games and Guided Imagery

Tools for Mental Health and School Professionals Working with Children, Adolescents, and Their Families

Monit Cheung

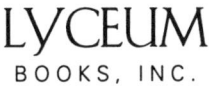

LYCEUM
BOOKS, INC.

Chicago, Illinois

© Lyceum Books, Inc., 2006

Published by

LYCEUM BOOKS, INC.
5758 S. Blackstone Ave.
Chicago, Illinois 60637
773+643-1903 (Fax)
773+643-1902 (Phone)
lyceum@lyceumbooks.com
http://www.lyceumbooks.com

10 9 8 7 6 5 4 3 2 1

ISBN: 0-925065-94-3

Figures 3, 5, 6, and 7 contain artwork by Mary Wu. Reprinted with permission.

Library of Congress Cataloging-in-Publication Data

Cheung, Monit.
   Therapeutic games and guided imagery : tools for mental health and school professionals : working with children, adolescents, and their families / Monit Cheung. — 1st ed.
      p. cm.
   Includes bibliographical references and index.
   ISBN 0-925065-94-3 (alk. paper)
   1. Play therapy. 2. Child psychotherapy. 3. Psychotherapy. 4. Games—Therapeutic use. I. Title.
RJ505.P6C54 2006
615.8'5153—dc22

   2005037274

Contents

Therapeutic Exercises

Part B Guided Imagery

For Children and Adolescents

For Families and Groups

Table of Functions

Therapeutic Games and Activities								
Icebreaker	A1	A2	A3	A7	A8	A13	A17	A20
	A22	A23	A24	A26	A27	A28	A34	A36
	A38	A39						
Rapport/relationship building	A1	A2	A4	A6	A7	A11	A14	A15
	A17	A19	A20	A22	A23	A24	A26	A27
	A28	A30	A31					
Assessment of functioning	A1	A2	A4	A6	A9	A10	A12	A14
	A15	A16	A18	A20	A21	A23	A24	A25
	A27	A29	A37					
Feelings expression	A3	A4	A5	A7	A8	A10	A11	A12
	A13	A14	A16	A17	A19	A21	A22	A25
	A26	A28	A29	A30	A31	A32	A33	A35
	A37	A38	A39					
Guided Imagery								
Concentration/awareness	B1	B3	B4	B7	B10	B13	B18	B19
	B22	B23	B24					
Visualization of success	B2	B4	B9	B11	B12	B15	B26	
Controlling anxiety	B2	B3	B5	B6	B8	B9	B11	B12
	B16	B20	B27					
Gaining insight	B2	B10	B14	B15	B17	B20	B21	B25
	B26	B28	B29	B30				

Preface

This book is a practice manual for social workers, counselors, school professionals, and other helping professionals in the medical and mental health fields. It provides a variety of therapeutic techniques for working with children and adolescents, individually or in family and small-group settings. This collection of thirty-nine therapeutic games and thirty guided imagery exercises was created and tested by a group of social workers and counseling psychologists under my guidance. It includes innovative ideas and empirically tested methods that aim to help clients achieve the maximum effect of psychotherapy in a short time.

The overall purpose of these therapeutic techniques is to assist clinicians in observing and assessing their clients' problems or issues, while helping clients relax, express their feelings, and enhance their ability to improve interpersonal relationships. In addition, clients are encouraged to regularly apply appropriately chosen relaxation exercises to reduce stress, so that they may develop a self-directed ritual that promotes better mental health. Clients learn how to use their five senses to search for peace, to ease their minds, and to find helpful insights to resolve personal problems.

The book presents two brief creative modalities in clinical practice. The first is a collection of therapeutic games and activities designed to help clients break their resistance to therapy, express their feelings, and join the therapist or group members in treatment activities. The second is a collection of guided imagery exercises to help clients relax when dealing with their problems or crises, and to work toward their therapeutic goals. Using these modalities in therapy can help children and adolescents, as well as their parents and other adults, gain insight through creative movements while maximizing their therapeutic interactions. Through the use of games and activities, therapists can help their clients rebuild confidence and develop a new perspective when dealing with their interpersonal relationships.

These games and exercises also provide various ways to prepare children, adolescents, and their families for entering into a helping relationship with their therapist. The multiple relaxation strategies and insight-gaining methods can help therapists and clients meet different kinds of mental health needs. I use a holistic perspective to organize these various themes of creative techniques; they include physical and mental relaxation, tension reduction, joining in an imagery journey, group involvement, connecting with nature, body-mind connections, and connections through insightful music in a guided imagery context.

This book has two parts: therapeutic games and activities, and guided imagery exercises. Each part is divided into a section for children and adolescents and one for families and groups. Since these activities and exercises were originally designed for individuals *or* for groups, they were divided for practical applications, but it should be noted that many can be used in either setting. This structure aims to promote maximum clinician flexibility and creativity; many of the exercises can be modified in vocabulary or content within these groups in order to suit individual client needs or preferences. Clinicians who wish to select exercises based on a specific mental disorder or social issue should consult table 2 (pp. 5–7) and table 3 (pp. 144–145). These tables cross-reference the primary functions of the activities with the assessment/treatment focus. At the end of the book, the index also cross-references all the exercises.

This text is intended to augment professional therapeutic training, and students should note that these exercises are not a shortcut to developing sound clinical skills and judgment. Clinical skills such as assessment, rapport building, and treatment planning are imperative for these exercises to be successful in a therapeutic context.

All of the creative ideas published in this book are based on clinical experiences and practical insights. The contributors wish to acknowledge their colleagues and clients for providing helpful suggestions in the creation and testing processes. Games and guided imagery exercises should be chosen *with* the clients, that is, not determined solely by the social worker, therapist, or practitioner.

Practitioners may use the materials from this book to meet the therapeutic needs of their clients. For other purposes, please write to the publisher to obtain formal approval. If you prerecord the guided imagery exercises for clients, please acknowledge the contributors and provide the following reference on the tape: *Therapeutic games and guided imagery: Tools for mental health and school professionals working with children, adolescents, and their families.* Edited by Monit Cheung. Published 2006 by Lyceum Books, Chicago.

Introduction

Theoretical Framework

Supporting the Use of Therapeutic Exercises

This book is organized into two parts: Therapeutic Games and Activities, and Guided Imagery. The inclusion of these creative and kinetic approaches to work with children, adolescents, and their families is based on the integrative practice framework built by the editor through an integration of her thirty years of clinical experiences in the fields of psychotherapy, counseling, and social work practice. This integrative framework supports the theoretical foundation of using alternative energy-generating approaches that supplement traditional talk therapy. Therapy is most effective if clients can integrate and use their kinetic senses to generate energy and uncover unused strengths for healing.

Figure 1 demonstrates how the integrated practice framework develops through an evidence-based understanding of the child's world. It also shows three major streams of theoretical supports—internal/external views, theory-based pointers, and the triadic energy of thinking-feeling-acting responsibilities. This framework starts with the influential factors, both internal and external, that affect our lives and behaviors. Internal factors come mainly from the instinctual and hereditary development of personality, while external factors occur in ecological systems, such as families, schools, peer relations, societal culture, religious and belief systems, the socioeconomic system, and the cultural and political environment. Practitioners with an integrative approach in clinical practice apply both internal and external analyses in working with their clients, both children and adults, according to their formative experiences. Such experiences, including observations made during direct or indirect contact with others in daily life and social interactions, can be meaningfully or traumatically accumulative, and in turn affect the individual's psychological reactions to situations and crises. Integrated in this practice framework is a group of theories from both the internal view and the external perspective. Psychoanalytic theories (see Caruth, 1988; Polusny & Follette, 1996) support the use of free association in games and guided imagery exercises to allow past experiences to surface. This process can bring the unconscious to an observable level, leading to client insight and helping practitioners identify appropriate strategies of therapy. Free association can also lead to discussions of the client's thinking patterns, which stem from the client's interpretations of

Fig. 1 The child's world

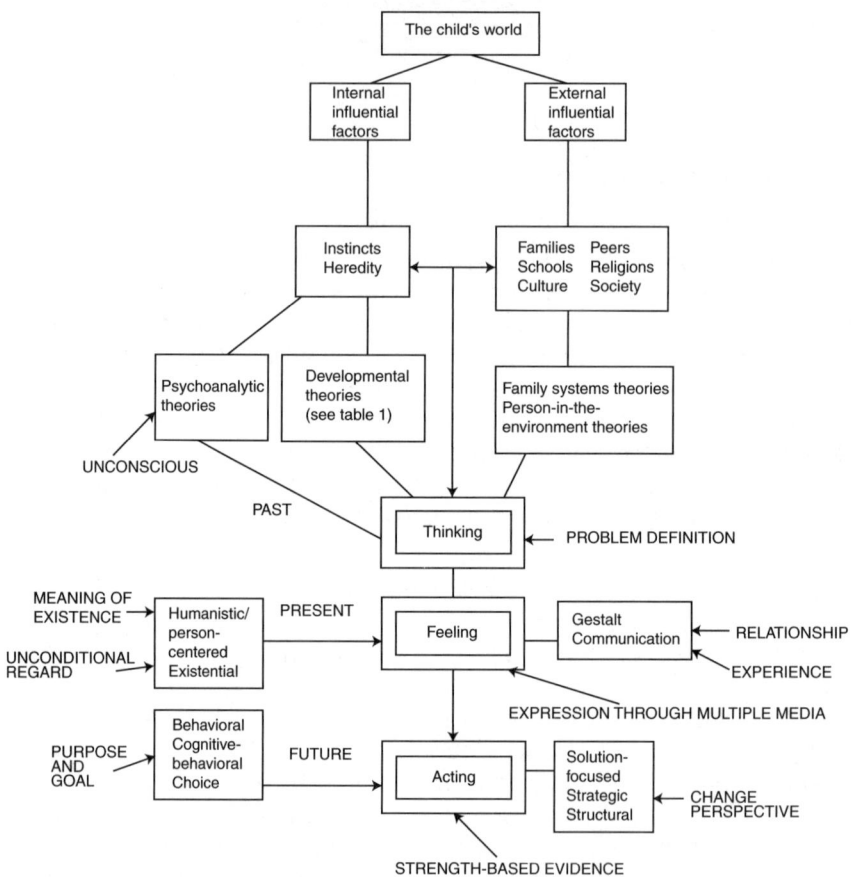

the reactions, comments, and behavior of others. From the external view, the second set of theories involves the social systems. Person-in-the-environment and family systems theories (Goldenberg & Goldenberg, 2004) present ideas about involving other people in the assessment process. In order to assess the cognitive and social functioning of an individual, the therapist must understand the interaction patterns among family members, and obtain a sense of the definition of the family in relation to other social systems such as peers, church, and cultural expectations. From an internal perspective, another category of theories is developmentally based. These theories include Erik Erikson's psychosocial development (1950), Sigmund Freud's psychosexual development (1975), Lawrence Kohlberg's moral development (1981), Margaret Mahler's early attachment development (McDevitt & Settlage, 1971), Abraham Maslow's hierarchy of needs (Lowry, 1973), and Jean Piaget's cognitive development (Murray, 2000). Each developmental theory explains an aspect of children's developmental tasks, including psychological, social, sexual, moral, attachment, basic but complex needs, language, and cognitive development. These eight major developmental tasks are embedded in each of the suggested games or exercises in order to maximize use of clients' energy and strengths. A summary of these theories in reference to periods of child development is provided in table 1. Clients' views are greatly influenced by developmental tasks through childhood, adolescence, and adulthood, and this summary provides a quick reference guide for therapists as they assist clients in achieving their therapeutic goals.

Erik Erikson's theories explain the development of trust, autonomy, initiative power, industrious energy, self-identity, and intimacy throughout childhood and adolescence. It is imperative to consider these tasks when designing a game or exercise for the client, as they will direct the practitioner in establishing a clear goal for therapy. For example, a toddler with separation anxiety will be guided to establish trust and learn the meaning of autonomy through selected therapeutic exercises. This psychosocial approach relates somatic changes to maturation, environmental resources, life changes, and life habits while providing explanations about how developmental movements can be related to unexpected changes (Newman & Newman, 2003). Utilizing this stage approach as a guide, table 1 cross-references the developmental stages with other theoretical discoveries of childhood growth and development. With the exception of the theories developed by Sigmund Freud and Abraham Maslow, the selected theories stress the importance of childhood development with an assumption that developmental tasks continue through adulthood.

These six theories are selected as the theoretical basis because they share a common thrust of identifying major developmental tasks and using each step as a reference point for goal setting, as well as for assessment and treatment. Sigmund Freud's psychosexual developmental stages for children include oral, anal, oedipal, latency, and puberty, and these stages provide guidance on how to assess clients' readiness to receive certain types of therapy. For example, if a therapist assesses that a child is fixated at a particular developmental stage, this child may benefit from engaging in games but may not receive the full therapeutic benefit of certain guided imagery exercises because he or she lacks certain developmental abilities.

Focusing on moral development, Lawrence Kohlberg (1981) identifies six stages to explain how children learn right from wrong and develop the skills of seeking clarification. Kohlberg does not seek to explain infant moral developmental stages, not necessarily because infants have not developed a moral sense, but because they do not have the language skills to identify their knowing or understanding. According to this theory, a typical child in play therapy can understand simple rules to be observed, followed by some explanations. With

Table 1 Exploring our personal world

Age of first development		Theory of human development					
Developmental period	Chronological age	Erikson's psychosocial development	Freud's psychosexual development	Kohlberg's moral development	Mahler's early attachment development	Maslow's hierarchy of needs	Piaget's cognitive development
Infancy	0–4 months	Trust vs. mistrust	Oral		Symbiotic stage	Physiological safety & security	Sensorimotor
	5–7 months			*Preconventional*	Hatching stage	Association, love, connectedness (with significant adults)	
	8–16 months		Anal	Stage 1 (reward or punishment)	Practicing stage		
	17–24 months	Autonomy vs. shame, doubt		Stage 2 (self or loved ones)			
Toddlerhood	2 years		Oedipal		Rapproachment		Preoperational (egocentric, memorization)
	3 years	Initiative vs. guilt			Object constancy		
Early-school age	4 years			*Conventional* Stage 3 (authority's approval)		Connectedness (with peers), social approval	
	5 years			Stage 4 (laws)			

Developmental period	Age					
Middle-school age	6–12 years	Industry vs. inferiority	Latency		Esteem, curiosity, recognition, character	Concrete operations (reversibility, sequencing)
Early adolescence	12–18 years	Identity vs. identity diffusion	Puberty	*Postconventional* Stage 5 (cooperative collaboration) Stage 6 (ethical principles)	Intellectual stimulation, creativity, competency	Formal operations (hypothesis testing, abstracting)
Later adolescence	18–22 years	Intimacy vs. isolation			Aesthetics, beauty	
Early adulthood	22–34 years	Generativity vs. self-absorption	Genitality		Order, symmetry of nature, devotion beyond self	
Middle adulthood	34–65 years	Integrity vs. disgust, despair				
Later adulthood	65+ years					

Note: Most theorists do not offer specific ages for the stages but include only a general range of developmental periods.

guided support, a child's moral senses can be discovered and expressed along with the utilization of appropriate skills learned in social interactions.

In recent neuropsychological research, brain development during the first three years of life is the most essential theoretical underpinning to understanding children's behaviors (Starting Points, 1994), especially when visual and auditory tools are applied to stimulate children's learning (Moughty, 2005). Margaret Mahler suggests that attachment and object constancy are the most crucial elements in establishing cohesive parent-child relationships (Mahler, Pine, & Bergman, 1975). Without a meaningful attachment to a parent figure during the early stages of development, a child must learn from games and other social activities, to find alternative ways to retain a healthy sense of belonging. According to Abraham Maslow, this need is associated with the need for safety, security, association, and connectedness. In a therapeutic setting, it is important to assess whether basic needs have been fulfilled before setting up therapeutic goals. With strong physical development, a child can connect with others through a milieu of physical movements, language usage, and feeling expressions. This kinetic connection is also based on Jean Piaget's theory that a person must learn to move, think, feel, and then test reasoning. Cognitive development is correlated to the successful achievement of one's sensorimotor skills during the early infancy stages. In childhood stages, language development is one of the essential steps to connect the thinking, feeling, and reasoning functions within an individual, and language expression is used to link these functions through social activities to connect this individual to the larger environment.

In addition to the internal perspective as presented in figure 1, kinetic movement orientation also has a theoretical base for clinical practice. Because psychotherapy cannot be completed without the expression of ideas, thoughts, feelings, and actions, language development is defined in this framework as the progressive use of multidimensional communication media including verbal and nonverbal, expressive and kinetic. In other words, for clients who may not see a "talking cure" as the only effective way of expressing frustrations or problems, language should include all types of verbal and nonverbal media, as well as physical movements. Assuming that talking is one of these communication tools, this framework in figure 1 addresses our lives by analyzing three major process-oriented responsibilities, namely, thinking, feeling, and acting (Corey, 2005). The accomplishment of these responsibilities determines how we analyze our problems, what experiences we use for this analysis, and when and how we act based on what we know. The analysis of our thinking is based on past experiences, while our experiential feelings affect our reactions toward crises or sudden changes that these experiences bring forth. Meanwhile, these thinking and feeling patterns determine our behavior or actions.

Our clients will express feelings when they have the opportunity to explore the meaning of life and existence through the therapeutic guidance of a humanistic and existential framework. Our clients will also discover their strengths and purpose in life after they have broken through resistance to change. Through games and guided movements in activating feelings, thoughts, and actions, they will be equipped with a true sense of ownership in creating and implementing solutions. With appropriate guidance, well-designed games and guided exercises allow practitioners to observe and work with clients in a natural social environment where typical interactions occur.

Explaining and Establishing the Goals and Roles of Therapeutic Exercises

Ten theories are summarized here to highlight the broad theoretical basis for creative therapy. Although early play therapy focused on the psychosocial and psychosexual developmental theories, creative therapies are supported by a variety of behavioral theories, including psychoanalytic, humanistic and person-centered, existential, gestalt, communication, behavioral, reality, structural, strategic, and solution-focused. Each selected theory has a unique set of assumptions to help practitioners plan theory-based goals of intervention and establish the role of creative therapeutic techniques.

The psychoanalytic and psychodynamic theories assume that reliving the past is the most natural means to uncover the long-buried unconscious, and that both the client and the practitioner can gain insight from past events to open a thought-generating process. The theoretical foundation is based on clinical observations that internal motivation is the impetus that moves a person to active thinking. Psychoanalytically speaking, the ultimate goal of games and exercises is to enhance the power of self-consciousness and to extract problem-solving energy from within a person toward the surface. The key is utilization of the client's past-oriented thinking to stimulate current therapeutic insight. Although the practitioner may keep professional interpretations in mind, the theoretical base of using games and guided imagery should be client-driven, not focused on the therapist's suggestions or personal judgment.

After processing the past, the suggested therapeutic exercises can also be used to process current feelings and relationships. This present-focused approach is supported by the here-and-now concepts derived from humanistic, person-centered, existential, gestalt, and communication theories (Goldenberg & Goldenberg, 2004; Satir, 1972). It assumes that personality is shaped by how an individual's image is projected through other people's comments. The creation of a "looking-glass self" through the professional provides a safe medium for the individual to express his or her feelings. The key is the creation of an encouraging and nurturing environment that allows for maximizing self-awareness for personal growth and relationship building.

The past and the present cannot stand alone without looking into the future. The third category of theories supporting these therapeutic exercises is the future-oriented approaches, including behavioral, reality, structural, strategic, and solution-focused theories. Futurist therapies are action focused with a goal. These theories support the idea that each game or exercise should have a goal (or a set of goals). Goal fulfillment gives meaning to the game to make it therapeutic. Each of these theories identifies the need to assess the problem, focus on the goal, and evaluate its outcomes. With a strong behaviorally driven plan, the client can enjoy his or her self-directed journey toward healing, with or without the presence of the therapist. The key to success is a committed, goal-setting process to empower clients and facilitate change.

This theoretical summary is by no means an exhaustive or complete description of the complex theoretical foundation for creative modalities. However, it does illustrate how the flexible use of past, present, and future orientations combine to help a client or family resolve internal or interpersonal conflicts. In addition, it helps practitioners understand the effectiveness of incorporating thinking, feeling, and acting into a holistic helping process. For a more comprehensive exploration of theoretical foundations of creative therapies, see the additional resources listed at the end of this book.

Here is a summary of the ten theories.

I. Psychoanalytic theory

   A. Assumptions

      1. Personality developed before birth and has developed further since birth.

      2. Id, ego, and superego govern our behavior and personality development.

      3. Failure to acquire either ego or superego functions is postulated to cause serious psychological disturbances, such as autism or schizophrenia.

      4. Defense mechanisms are used to protect the self.

   B. Goals of intervention

      1. To develop or revise the psychic structures and functions in order to foster optimum development.

      2. To make the unconscious conscious through the use of interpretations.

      3. To promote self-awareness of behavioral changes through insight.

   C. Roles of therapeutic exercises

      1. To establish rapport within the child's world.

      2. To observe clients and to gather information about clients' physical and social functioning.

      3. To communicate with clients at the clients' level.

II. Humanistic and person-centered theory

    A. Assumptions

        1. Clients' mere presence in the play-therapy environment is therapeutic and meaningful.

        2. Children, adolescents, and family members of any developmental level can engage in play.

        3. Relationships between the therapist and the client are of utmost importance.

    B. Goals of intervention

        1. To provide an optimum environment with clients that allows for the development of self-actualization.

        2. To provide a positively reinforcing environment to reduce tension and conflict.

        3. To understand clients' perspective(s) through empathic communication.

        4. To help clients resolve internal conflict through understanding of their feelings.

    C. Roles of therapeutic exercises

        1. To build a warm and friendly relationship with clients.

        2. To bring out the real self of clients.

        3. To help clients establish an atmosphere of permissiveness in a natural environment.

        4. To maintain respect for clients' ability to solve their problems.

        5. To uncover clients' strengths (and weaknesses, if necessary).

        6. To communicate.

III. Existential theory

    A. Assumptions

        1. Each individual has a set of unique characteristics.

        2. Choice, freedom, responsibility, and self-determination are important elements in life.

        3. We are the authors of our lives, and we re-create ourselves through our projects.

    B. Goals of intervention

        1. To help clients understand that they are free, so that they can become aware of their possibilities.

2. To challenge clients to recognize the ramifications of their actions and behaviors.

3. To identify responsibilities that accompany our freedom to choose.

C. Roles of therapeutic exercises

1. To increase clients' self-awareness.

2. To allow clients to give their own interpretations.

3. To observe clients' current experience.

IV. Gestalt theory

A. Assumptions

1. Individuals are responsible for their own behavior and experience.

2. Participating in an experiential approach, clients come to grips with what they are feeling, thinking, and doing.

3. Clients have the capacity to do their own seeing, feeling, sensing, and interpreting.

B. Goals of intervention

1. To help clients relax and regain self-support.

2. To assist clients in gaining self-awareness.

C. Roles of therapeutic exercises

1. To confront clients in a nonthreatening way.

2. To role-play or imagine all the significant parts in a client's life.

3. To observe clients' nonverbal behaviors.

V. Communication theory

A. Assumptions

1. Relationships are established through proper communication.

2. Fear of rejection is a threat to self-concept.

3. A nurturing environment is necessary to promote self-worth.

B. Goals of intervention

1. To find and establish a supportive environment.

2. To enhance individual growth and development.

C. Roles of therapeutic exercises

1. To allow clients to express themselves in a relaxed environment.

2. To understand the various roles a child or adolescent plays in the family.

3. To observe communication styles.

4. To encourage interpersonal communication.

VI. Behavioral and cognitive-behavioral theory

    A. Assumptions

        1. Human behaviors are learned and can be unlearned.

        2. Behaviors and thinking patterns are connected.

        3. Play and relaxation techniques are applicable for individuals in all developmental stages.

    B. Goals of intervention

        1. To discover patterns of reinforcements, consequences, and cognition that shape and maintain clients' developmentally inappropriate behavior and then help clients alter them.

        2. To model appropriate behaviors through limit setting and structured therapeutic sessions.

    C. Roles of therapeutic exercises

        1. To provide a natural means to observe clients' behaviors and uncover clients' thinking patterns.

        2. To produce a nonthreatening environment in which to test reinforcement schedules.

        3. To evaluate progress and changes.

VII. Choice theory

    A. Assumptions

        1. A person behaves in a certain way to reach a purpose.

        2. All individuals need to love and be loved, and all individuals need to feel worthwhile to themselves and to others.

        3. Negative reinforcement is not suitable for bringing about change.

    B. Goals Intervention

        1. To teach parents and their children strategies for meeting their own needs responsibly.

        2. To uncover and maximize clients' potential to meet their basic needs in socially appropriate and responsible ways.

    C. Roles of therapeutic exercises

        1. To uncover clients' needs.

        2. To understand clients' experiences of unmet needs.

        3. To communicate and model responsible behaviors.

B. Goals of intervention

    1. To reconstruct new realities that would allow clients to make productive choices.

    2. To identify clients' strengths and resources.

    3. To identify what has worked in the past.

C. Roles of therapeutic exercises

    1. To search for exceptions to a complaint through play.

    2. To amplify clients' spontaneous suggestions for solutions through natural means of communication.

    3. To validate clients' experience.

Forms and Instruments

Drawing Our Feelings

Expression of feelings is the most popular psychotherapeutic procedure. Figure 2 is a form I use in addressing the client's feelings and assessing the client's progress in the counseling process. Since many therapeutic games are used for assessing, exploring, and treating clients' emotional traumas, a sheet with thirty-two feeling faces (fig. 3) is included here. It may help practitioners design games and assist clients in identifying their feelings. Unlike other drawings of feeling faces, this sheet is unique in the following aspects: (1) it identifies fifteen "positive" feelings, feelings that are socially acceptable and desirable, and fifteen "difficult" feelings, feelings that are stress-related or negatively impact the client; (2) fifteen faces are female and fifteen are male; (3) the hair styles reflect various ethnic backgrounds (Asian, Caucasian, Hispanic, African American); and (4) two unidentified feelings are included to allow for clients' unique input. These feeling faces are organized in alphabetical order of the feeling words, and therefore they are mixed in terms of "positive" and "difficult" feelings.

For the convenience of game creation and immediate practical use, five sheets are provided in this workbook (figs. 3–7): (1) feeling faces with the associated feeling words, (2) feeling words without the feeling faces, (3) feeling faces without the feeling words, (4) difficult feelings only, and (5) positive feelings only. These faces can be cut out and pasted on index cards for designing therapeutic games described in this book. Practitioners can also use these sheets to create their own therapeutic games, such as matching, Go Fish, guessing games, Chutes and Ladders, and so forth. Remember to remind clients that no feelings are "wrong" feelings, and to reassure them that all feelings have validity and functional means of expression. Take care not to react negatively to the expression of unpleasant or uncomfortable emotions.

In addition to game creation, these sheets can be used to help children and adolescents identify their feelings after completing a guided imagery exercise.

Fig. 2 A feeling exercise

We all have feelings. We can have more than one feeling at any given time. We can have mixed and confused feelings. We can have simple or complex feelings. Let's share our feelings today and then compare these feelings when we come to a closure later.

DRAW or WRITE.

Feelings Now	Feelings at Closure
Date _____	Date _____

Feeling Words

Angry, Anxious, Ashamed, Bored, Cheerful, Confident, Confused, Cool/Calm, Depressed, Disgusted, Ecstatic, Embarrassed, Enraged, Excited, Exhausted, Frightened, Great, Happy, Hilarious, Hopeful, Joyful, Lonely, Lovestruck, Mad, Okay, Relaxed, Sad, Satisfied, Shocked, Silly

Unknown? Let's explore.

Fig. 3 Feeling faces

Angry	Anxious	Ashamed	Bored
Cheerful	Confident	Confused	Cool/Calm
Depressed	Disgusted	Ecstatic	Embarrassed
Enraged	Excited	Exhausted	Frightened
Great	Happy	Hilarious	Hopeful
Joyful	Lonely	Lovestruck	Mad
Okay	Relaxed	Sad	Satisfied
Shocked	Silly	Unknown	Unknown

Fig. 4 Feeling faces, words only

Angry	Anxious	Ashamed	Bored
Cheerful	Confident	Confused	Cool/Calm
Depressed	Disgusted	Ecstatic	Embarrassed
Enraged	Excited	Exhausted	Frightened
Great	Happy	Hilarious	Hopeful
Joyful	Lonely	Lovestruck	Mad
Okay	Relaxed	Sad	Satisfied
Shocked	Silly	Unknown	Unknown

Fig. 5 Feeling faces, unlabeled

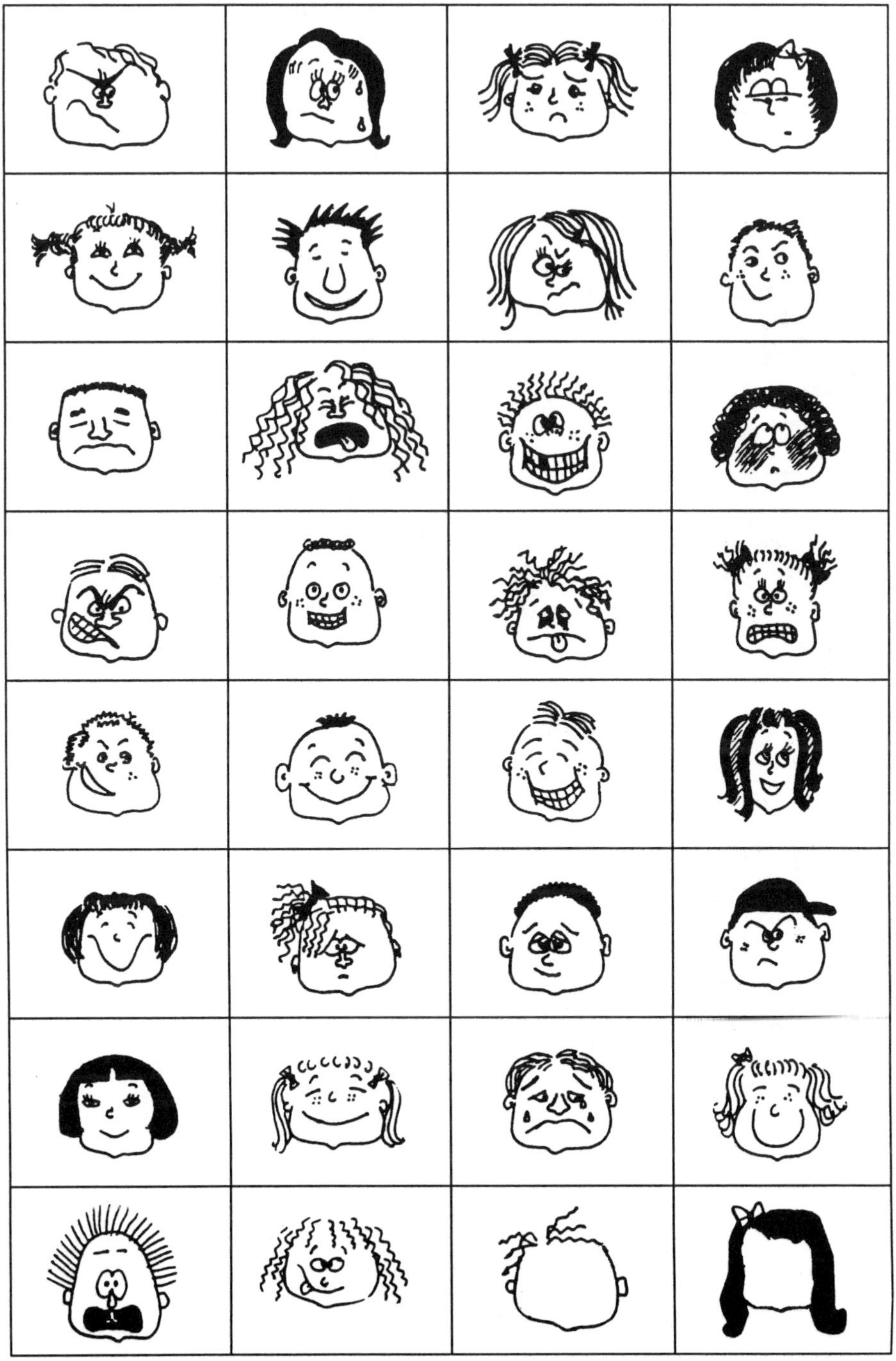

Fig. 6 Feeling faces, difficult feelings

Angry	Anxious	Ashamed
Bored	Confused	Depressed
Disgusted	Embarrassed	Enraged
Exhausted	Frightened	Lonely
Mad	Sad	Shocked

Fig. 7 Feeling faces, positive feelings

Cheerful	Confident	Cool/Calm
Ecstatic	Excited	Great
Happy	Hilarious	Hopeful
Joyful	Lovestruck	Okay
Relaxed	Satisfied	Silly

It is difficult to express in words how a person feels at the moment without any reference points. After implementing a relaxation exercise or a guided exercise, the therapist's first question may be, "How do you feel right now?" The client may use these feeling faces to identify feelings that result from the exercise.

Providing Observations

In addition to the feeling faces, two sets of observation forms are provided to help both practitioners and clients document and enhance behavioral changes. The first set of observation forms is designed for practitioners for use with children and adolescents during play therapy (fig. 8) or with family/group work (fig. 9). These forms contain ground rules and observation points to guide practitioners. The second set of forms is designed for clients to report on their own targeted behavioral changes. One form (fig. 10) is a behavioral modification chart for young children, focusing on simple and practical positive reinforcement techniques. The other form (fig. 11) is a family journal that provides a time-limited intervention for families to use at home. Self-directed behavioral changes are the ultimate goals after the implementation of guided therapeutic intervention. These tools are easy to use, brief, and intervention-focused, and can be modified to suit the needs of clients. For the games and exercises suggested in this book, these forms can help clients measure behavior changes and encourage clients to maintain a record of their self-directed assignments.

Fig. 8 Observation form for children and adolescents in play therapy

Name _____

Age _____

Caseworker _____

Ground Rules

1.   Set time limit (_____ minutes).

2.   Cannot hurt self or others.

3.   Put game pieces or toys in their original place.

4.   Others _____

     _____

Date	Game or activity	Participants	Time spent	Therapeutic goal (list each goal separately)	Mood observed	Feelings expressed	Evaluation (1 = not useful, 5 = very useful)
							1 2 3 4 5
							1 2 3 4 5
							1 2 3 4 5
							1 2 3 4 5
							1 2 3 4 5

Fig. 9 Observation form for families or groups

Name of identified patient _____ (Age ___; F or M)

Participant A _____(Age ___; F or M)

Participant B _____(Age ___; F or M)

Participant C _____(Age ___; F or M)

Participant D _____(Age ___; F or M)

Participant E _____(Age ___; F or M)

Caseworker _____

Ground Rules

1.   Set time limit (_____ minutes).

2.   Cannot hurt self or others.

3.   Put game pieces or toys in their original place.

4.   Others _____

    _____

Date	Game or activity	Participants	Time spent	Therapeutic goal (list each goal separately)	Mood observed	Feelings expressed	Evaluation (1 = not useful, 5 = very useful)
							1 2 3 4 5
							1 2 3 4 5
							1 2 3 4 5
							1 2 3 4 5
							1 2 3 4 5

Fig. 10 Behavioral modification schedule for young children

Child's name _____   Goal ___ (number) happy faces
Time frame _____ to _____   Anticipated award _____
Happy-face behaviors _____
      Happy-Face Behaviors

1	2	3	4	5
6	7	8	9	10
11	12	13	14	15
16	17	18	19	20
21	22	23	24	25
26	27	28	29	30

Mad-face behaviors _____
      Mad-Face Behaviors

-1	-2	-3	-4	-5
-6	-7	-8	-9	-10

Total scores at end of time frame _____
Recorded by _____ (child) and _____ (parent)

Fig. 11 Family journal

Participants

_____   _____
_____   _____
_____   _____

Time frame _____ to _____

An activity shared by the family each day

Examples   □ Spend ten minutes of quality time together
            □ Recite one daily affirmation statement together

Family Members' Initials (marked each day)

1	2	3	4	5
6	7	8	9	10
11	12	13	14	15
16	17	18	19	20
21	22	23	24	25
26	27	28	29	30

Part A
Therapeutic Games
and Activities

Introduction

According to choice theory, human beings need to realize a sense of achievement for their own growth and development, and often desire to have fun and enjoy themselves through the process of self-actualization (Glasser, 1998). Children love to play, and so do adults. However, we often neglect the importance of play in establishing adult-child relationships, believing that play belongs only to children. Consequently, adult-child interaction patterns become divided into two distinct spheres—the world of work for adults and the world of play for children. But in reality, work and play can be integrated for every client, especially in psychotherapy.

Psychologists have studied many aspects of human needs and have identified different theories to describe the process of human development (see figure 1 and table 1). It is important to note that the use of "play" in therapy does not involve only one behavioral theory, but is derived from a developmental perspective (Newman & Newman, 2003; Thompson & Rudolph, 2004; Webb, 1999).

Stages in Play Development

Hurlock (1972, p. 287) defines play as "*any* activity engaged in for the enjoyment it gives, without consideration of the end result." In play therapy, however, the end result requires significant consideration. Of equal importance is the process of play. Child development through play is an important criterion when an activity is being selected. Children develop their "play" skills through four stages—exploratory stage, toy stage, play stage, and daydream stage. Adults, on the other hand, integrate the concept "play" in their daily activities.

In the exploratory stage, children above three months old merely handle objects and make random movements. The toy stage begins in the first year and reaches a peak between seven and eight years. The play stage begins when children enter school. A variety of play activities such as games, sports, and hobbies are available to them. Playing with friends, schoolmates, relatives, and neighbors becomes an integral part of their social development. The last stage of play development involves daydreaming, pretending, and being creative. These different forms of mental play stimulate children's mental, cognitive, and moral development. People develop their creativity, or rigidity, through this developmental process. Adults often find that "playing" or "games" are not part of their vocabularies because these activities can be perceived as childish and immature. In therapy, however, play can be reframed as a channel of communication and a means of relaxation. Using creative means to help clients relax and communicate with one another is a way to encourage participation and stimulate discussions.

Applying this developmental aspect to play therapy, the practitioner can engage clients in games and activities while assessing the nature and extent of social and cognitive development. For example, preschool children like to be close to their caretakers in their play time to engage in the so-called mother games. Children aged five to eight engage in individual or solitary play. They play with others in practice games such as guessing and hide-and-seek, if they know their playmates well. Otherwise, they may spend time watching others and acting the part of the onlooker. Children aged eight to ten like to organize team games or games with rules that require competitive skills and regulations. Older children and adolescents (ages eleven to seventeen) as well as adults may enjoy individual or cooperative activities that do not require competition among the players. Engaging clients in age-appropriate activities gives them the opportunity to express themselves in a nonthreatening environment in which they feel comfortable and relaxed.

Applications

Games and activities often help children and adolescents enter a therapeutic relationship in a natural and nurturing way. Practical suggestions are included in each game or exercise. These experiential exercises can help clients find deeper meaning in their lives and gain insights into their personal world. However, it is important to note that these exercises may not suit every client. Careful selection, ongoing monitoring, and evaluation of outcomes are highly recommended.

Therapists may initially feel the need to approach these therapeutic games with a more directive approach: explaining the rules and parameters of the game, providing the materials, delineating a time frame for play, and redirecting any excessive digression from the activity. While directive approaches to therapeutic exercises certainly have merit, using more nondirective or client-directed approaches may help clients maximize their potential creativity. Ideally, therapists should eventually become comfortable applying both directive and nondirective approaches, so that they can evaluate clients therapeutically but not limit creativity or enjoyment.

Table 2 cross-references the assessment or treatment focus of each exercise with four broad functions of the games: icebreaker, rapport/relationship building, assessment of functioning, and feelings expression. Therapists may use this table as a guide; however, they should not feel limited by it. Many of the games can be modified to suit client needs and preferences.

Suggested Modifications

The first step of applying this workbook is to choose a game or exercise that contains a desirable purpose. The next step is to check the applicability of this game or exercise to a particular clientele. What makes these games and exercises unique is their flexibility and applicability, demonstrated by testing them in actual work with clients. In other words, modifications can be made to suit

Table 2. Therapeutic games by function and assessment/treatment focus

Game		Functions			Assessment/treatment focus
	Icebreaker	Rapport/relationship building	Assessment of functioning	Feelings expression	
A1	✓	✓	✓		ADHD
A2	✓	✓	✓		Depression, isolation, chronic illness (spina bifida)
A3	✓			✓	Sexual abuse, childhood trauma
A4		✓	✓	✓	Social inhibition, communication
A5				✓	Anger control
A6		✓	✓		Communication
A7	✓	✓		✓	Problem solving
A8	✓			✓	Mixed feelings
A9			✓		Adoption, foster home, grief
A10			✓	✓	Adoption, divorce, foster home
A11		✓		✓	Problem solving, terminal illness
A12			✓	✓	Sexual abuse, anger
A13	✓			✓	Communication
A14		✓	✓	✓	Coping strategies, sexual abuse
A15		✓	✓		Bullying

Table 2. (continued) **Therapeutic games by function and assessment/treatment focus**

Game	Icebreaker	Rapport/relationship building	Assessment of functioning	Feelings expression	Assessment/treatment focus
		Functions			
A16			✓	✓	Self-esteem, mixed feelings
A17	✓	✓		✓	Self-image, empower-ment, affirmation
A18			✓		Childhood trauma
A19		✓		✓	Adoption
A20	✓	✓	✓		Fears, concerns
A21			✓	✓	Life events
A22	✓	✓		✓	Self-awareness, relationships, self-esteem
A23	✓	✓	✓		Family connections
A24	✓	✓	✓		Family dynamics
A25			✓	✓	Divorce, grief
A26	✓	✓		✓	Processing feelings
A27	✓	✓	✓		Free association
A28	✓	✓		✓	Problem disclosure
A29			✓	✓	Problem identification, eating disor-der, divorce
A30		✓		✓	Communi-cation
A31		✓		✓	Self-image
A32				✓	Grief
A33				✓	Mixed feelings

Table 2. (continued) **Therapeutic games by function and assessment/treatment focus**

Game	Icebreaker	Rapport/ relationship building	Assessment of functioning	Feelings expression	Assessment/ treatment focus
			Functions		
A34	✓				Problem identification, self-esteem
A35				✓	Anger, hyperactivity
A36	✓				Peer influences, goal setting
A37			✓	✓	Problem identification
A38	✓			✓	Communication
A39	✓			✓	Privacy

the needs of a specific client or family. Modifying the therapeutic games will assist practitioners in tailoring the therapeutic tools that are most relevant to the client's situation. Before modifying a game for a client, consider the following:

1. Developmental stage or abilities of the client
   - Will the language be too mature/immature as written?
   - Does the client have a firm grasp of the English language? If not, is it possible to modify the language or locate a suitable interpreter (not a family member) to assist without interfering with the therapeutic intervention?
   - Will the items in the game be easily understood?
   - Does the game require reading ability? At what level?
2. The therapeutic level for the client
   - Will an additional icebreaker be required before applying the game or exercise?
   - Will any language or items in the game be counterproductive to the therapeutic process?
   - Is closure required if the therapeutic purpose is achieved before the end of the game or exercise?

3. The client's gender, religion, and culture or ethnicity
   - Could this modification be interpreted as offensive or hostile?
   - Does this modification communicate that the therapist appreciates the client's innate dignity and worth?
   - Would the client be willing to assist in determining what to include or modify in the exercise based on his or her cultural background? Can the client assist the therapist in understanding his or her unique cultural or religious traditions?

After considering the above, use creativity in applying a modification. Here are some examples.

1. Use a game with a different age group than the one indicated.
   - Try Memory Chain (A32) with adults or older adolescents. If desired, clients can use different artistic media to make a more complex end product; for example, making a memory scrapbook with pictures accompanying the memories, or making a collage or mobile out of symbolic representations of the memories.
   - Try Deck of Feelings (A4) with adults, couples, or families. When appropriate, add feeling words to the list, based on their input.

2. Use a game with individuals with a different therapeutic issue than the one indicated.
   - Try Operational Anger Release (A12) with children frustrated by chronic medical conditions. Modify questions to reflect how they perceive the medical procedures.
   - Try Chinese Adoption (A19) with adopted children from another country, or start with symbol drawing and try the game with biracial children coping with identity issues.
   - Try Facing Divorce Feelings (A25) with a client dealing with any difficult situation, such as bullying at school or learning anxiety.

3. Use individual games with groups, and vice versa.
   - Try Floating through Changes (A9) and My "Family" Home (A10) in a family session with foster/adoptive/biological parents, siblings, and other caregivers.
   - Try using Sandy Feelings (A13) as a family exercise to express feelings of grief, anger, or sadness.
   - Try Journal of Feelings (A30) as an individual exercise to encourage clients to acknowledge the range of good and bad feelings they have throughout the week.

Therapeutic Games and Activities for Children and Adolescents

A1
ADHD Relaxation Game
Monit Cheung

Items Needed

A big soft die; copies of the blank "Right Foot" and "Left Foot" sheets as needed (figures A1.1, A1.2); a "Start" sheet and a "Good!" sheet (see figures A1.3, A1.4); 20–40 index cards (3" × 5"); game piece for each player; small prizes

Target Population

Children 3 to 6 with attention deficit or hyperactivity disorder

Children who need to learn how to relax before taking a test or doing a task

Purpose

To break the ice

To build rapport, encourage children to do things gently, and assess functioning

To educate children about the importance of concentration and relaxation

To systematically teach children to use relaxation techniques for concentration

Procedure

Before meeting with the player, create the "Right" cards. Put the word "Right" on an index card, and a suggested phrase on the other side (see table A1.1). Other phrases can be created to meet the player's needs.

Explain to the player that this game aims to teach how to concentrate and relax, and that it is important to practice concentration and relaxation. Tell the player to concentrate on the game and nothing else, and not to disrupt or destroy any object in the room, including the foot sheets.

Ask the player to take off his or her shoes and draw both feet on two sheets of paper, the right foot on one and the left foot on the other. The drawing of the feet can be used as a relaxation rehearsal. Prompt the player to draw slowly and carefully. The therapist can make copies of at least twenty pairs of feet for this exercise. Use the copies of the "Right Foot" and "Left Foot" sheets as necessary to ensure forty foot sheets in total.

Begin to position the sheets on the floor to form a circle. Begin with the "Start" sheet. Then, moving counterclockwise, place a "Left Foot" sheet next, then a "Right Foot" sheet, a "Left Foot" sheet, and so on. Continue alternating left and right sheets to form a circle that uses all of the foot sheets. If applied in a group setting, the foot sheets from the different players do not necessarily need to be placed next to each other. Complete the circle with the "Good!" sheet next to the "Start" sheet. After all the sheets are in place, write a number (from 1 to 40 for the twenty pairs of feet) on each of the sheets to help the player count. Place "Right" cards in the center of the circle.

Explain to the player that he or she will now learn how to do deep breathing to relax. Practice a few deep breaths with the player. Begin the game by allowing the player to choose a game piece and place it on the "Start" sheet. Before beginning a turn, ask the player to take a deep breath. The player should then throw the die and advance the game piece the number of spaces indicated. If the game piece lands on a "Right Foot" sheet, then the player will draw a "Right" card from the center of the circle, read the instructions on the card, and perform the activity indicated.

After landing on or passing the "Good!" sheet for the first time, the game piece will be replaced by the player. In this round, the player will first take two deep breaths before throwing the die. The player will then walk gently on the sheets with the appropriate feet, that is, the player should place his or her right foot on the "Right Foot" sheet and left foot on the "Left Foot" sheet. Remind the player that relaxation and concentration can maintain the sheets in good shape while walking on them. (*Caution:* If children do not seem ready to walk on the sheets after the first round, continue using the game pieces.)

The game can end at any time. When the player seems to lose interest in the game or can no longer focus, lead some deep breathing exercises, and ask the player to take turns reading the "Right" cards. Prizes may be used to reinforce appropriate behaviors, such as following the instructions.

Function in Assessment and Treatment

Assessment

This exercise can be used as an assessment tool to evaluate the concentration level of the child. It can also serve as an introduction activity for children to learn deep breathing techniques. Children with ADHD usually have a hard time following instructions. This game can help these children associate following instructions with enjoying themselves. Refrain from using negative reinforcement or punishment during this activity.

Treatment

Use this game in individual treatment sessions to demonstrate appropriate behavior and suggest strategies for concentration. The child can identify his or her problems in performing the exercise, and you and the child can talk about ways to improve. A reinforcement chart can be used with the activity. A sticker or happy face can be the reward for a successful game. This can help the child relate positive reinforcement with appropriate behaviors.

Try these follow-up questions to assess progress.

1. Show me an example of "appropriate" or "good" behavior.
2. Have you shown this kind of behavior in the past week? When and where did you show it?
3. What did other people (such as your parents or teachers) say when you showed your "good" behavior?
4. Show me an example of "inappropriate" or "bad" behavior.
5. Have you shown this kind of behavior in the past week? When and where did you show it?
6. When you were walking in the past week, did you try the concentration method we did together to stay focused? If not, let's practice once more today.

Fig. A1.1 Left-foot outline

Left Foot

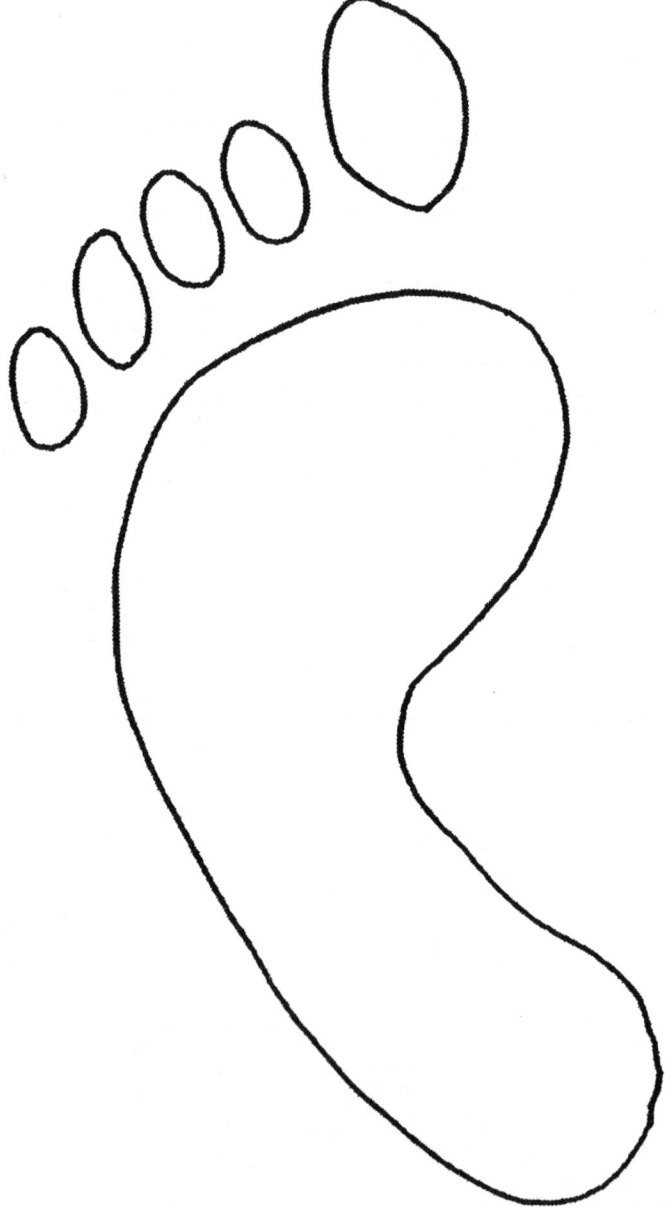

Fig. A1.2 Right-foot outline

Right Foot

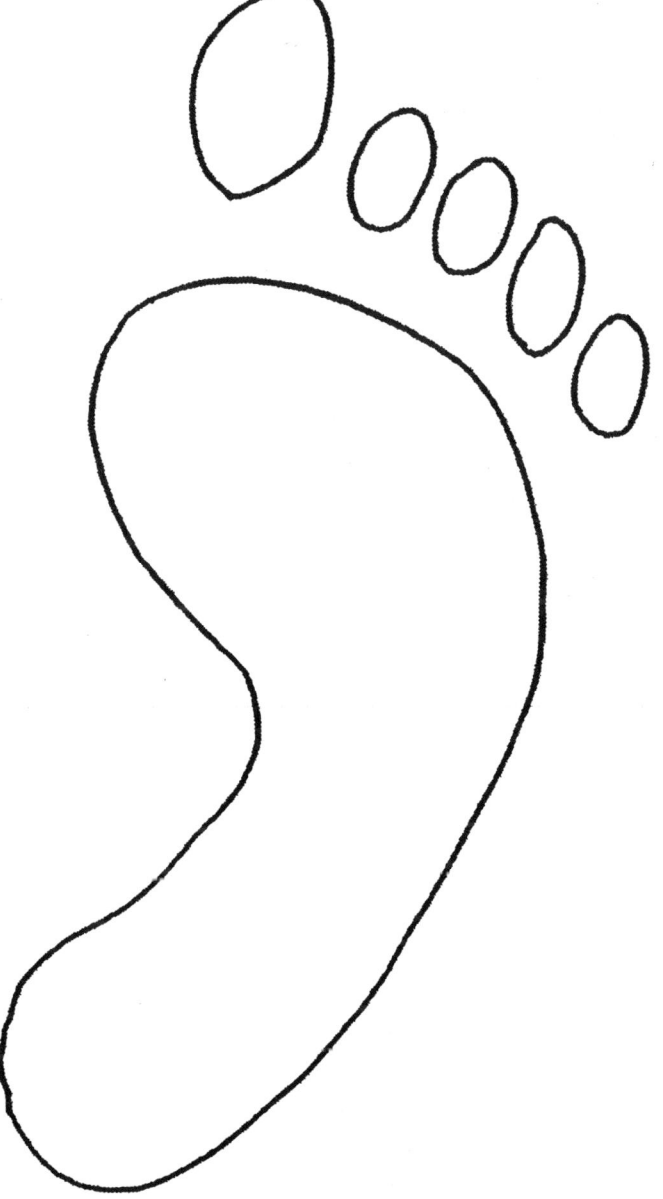

Fig. A1.3 Start card

START

1

Fig. A1.4 Praise card

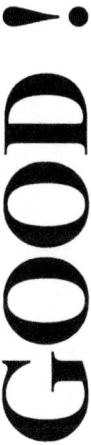

Table A1.1 Phrases for Right cards

Say, "Concentration" 3 times as slowly as you can.	You won a prize! Say, "Great!"
Clap your hands 3 times as softly as you can.	Take a deep breath and say, "Thank you!"
Count from 1 to 3 as slowly as you can.	Close your eyes and say, "I am relaxed!"
Close your eyes and count from 1 to 5.	Close your eyes and take a deep breath.
Imagine you are a feather. Do a slow and soft movement.	Imagine you are a flower. Make your hands like the petals.
Say, "I am great!" 3 times as gently as you can.	Say, "Quiet, please" very quietly.
Say to one of us, "Hi, how are you?"	Say, "Hello" 3 times as softly as you can.
Raise your hands as high as you can.	Say, "Good-bye" 3 times politely.
Close your eyes and say, "I am wonderful!"	Say, "Good!" 3 times as softly as you can.
Raise your shoulders to your ears and say, "Good!"	Take 3 breaths as deeply as you can.
Yawn 3 times and say, "Good!"	Laugh 3 times. Say, "I am having fun."
Smile at one of us and hold your smile for 3 seconds.	Say, "Relaxed" 3 times and stand very still.
You won a prize! Say, "Thank you!"	You won a prize! Say, "Hooray!"

A2

Ask Me

Kelli L. Beveridge

Items Needed

30 index cards (3" × 5") with therapeutic questions from table A2.1; pen or marker

Target Population

Children 6 to 12 with chronic illnesses, such as spina bifida

Purpose

To break the ice

To build rapport

To assess children in a short time for psychosocial problems or problems with medical regimen related to spina bifida (or other chronic illnesses)

Procedure

Ask the child if he or she would like to play a short game with you so you can catch up on how he or she is doing since the last visit. Show the child the cards, mix them up, and briefly explain how you both will take turns answering the questions on the cards by saying the first thing that comes to mind. You could answer from the perspective of other children with similar illnesses.

Go through as many cards as needed to assess the child for depression, isolation, and problems with regimen compliance.

Use a sticker or a small gift to encourage participation.

If the child is willing, create new cards with the child.

Function in Assessment and Treatment

Assessment

This game is rooted in choice-theory principles. Children with spina bifida tend to have developmental delays and chronic problems with medical regimen compliance. They also tend to be socially isolated, particularly at school. This game helps you assess these problem areas, in addition to assessing if there is an adverse dependency between the parent(s) and the child. This game can be modified for those with profound developmental delays or other kinds of chronic illnesses, such as those who require IV treatments, blood tests, or physical therapy. Modify questions according to client needs.

Treatment

The child will learn that it is OK to talk about his or her feelings in a safe and nurturing environment. After the game, work on problem solving with the child and/or parent(s) to help the family take steps to ensure that the child achieves independence and social involvement. Discuss progress with the family during subsequent visits to ascertain what steps the family has taken to assist the child in building self-esteem and becoming more involved with others.

Therapeutic questions are divided into three major categories: specific questions dealing with spina bifida, questions probing for signs of denial and depression, and general questions designed to establish rapport and to assess current levels of isolation and socialization (table A2.1).

Table A2.1 Therapeutic questions

Spina bifida

1. Are there any other kids that you know at school (or in the hospital) who have spina bifida (or other illness)?

2. What do you think is the most uncomfortable part of learning how to cath?

3. Name at least one thing that you can do at home without your parents' help.

4. Do you feel comfortable with the nurses who cath you when you are at school?

5. What is one thing you don't like about having spina bifida?

6. Who is your favorite person in your family (who helps you cath)?

7. How do you feel about the cathing and bowel program?

8. Do you feel ready to give cathing a try?

9. How do you feel about coming to the clinic/hospital?

10. Name at least one new task that you've tried in the last two weeks, without your family's help.

Table A2.1 (continued) **Therapeutic questions**

Depression/denial

1. What do you do when you feel angry?

2. What is the most embarrassing thing that has ever happened to you?

3. Do you laugh a lot? Let's laugh together.

4. Do you like to act silly sometimes? Let's act silly for a few seconds.

5. What do you do when you feel sad?

6. Whom in your family do you like to talk to the most when you are feeling sad?

7. What kinds of things annoy you or make you feel sad?

8. What was the happiest day of your life?

9. How do you feel when you see someone do something that you can't do because of your illness?

10. Do your mother and father ask you to try doing more things on your own—like brushing your teeth, getting dressed, or helping out around the house?

Socialization/isolation

1. Do you like to participate in sports with other kids who have disabilities?

2. Have you ever thought of what you'd like to be when you grow up?

3. What is one of your favorite toys or hobbies?

4. What do you enjoy doing the most with your family?

5. Who are some of the friends you play with at school?

6. What are some of the things that you like to do with your friends?

7. What was the best Christmas (or other holiday/occasion) gift you ever received?

8. Do you have a best friend?

9. If you had three wishes, what would you wish for?

10. What are your favorite TV shows?

Cartoon-Story Game

Alyssa I. Sanders

Items Needed

A piece of construction paper (12" × 18") for each player; assorted crayons

Target Population

Children 4 and up and adolescents who have been abused

Adults with childhood trauma

All cultures and socioeconomic backgrounds

Purpose

To break the ice

To help children or adults express themselves

Procedure

Draw eight cartoon boxes on a piece of construction paper. The paper can be folded into eighths and then outlined with a crayon (see fig. A3.1).

Ask the participant to draw a cartoon story using crayons. The participant should number the drawings from 1 to 8 to show the sequence of events.

After the participant finishes the cartoons, ask him or her to tell or share the story corresponding to the pictures.

In groups, allow participants to pass if they do not wish to share their story. Put a sticker on the picture to symbolize that the participant has not yet shared this section of his or her story. You could also give a token to the client to remind him or her that this part of the story can be shared at a later time.

Function in Assessment and Treatment

Assessment

This game gives clients an opportunity to express themselves through creative illustrations. The structured nature of the cartoon enables clients to tell a story, while allowing them to use their imagination. The game may be used as an icebreaker in individual or group counseling. If you use the cartoon story in an individual counseling session with a younger child, you may want to take part in the exercise and draw a cartoon as well. Sharing your story may help build trust with the child. This game may also help clients tell stories that they may not be comfortable articulating aloud. As always, use caution in sexual abuse cases.

Treatment

Use the client's story as a guideline for more probing questions. For example, ask the client how a cartoon character feels at a particular point in the story or ask questions such as, "How do you know what the rabbit wants to do? How do you know he feels sad?" If helpful, the cartoon story can be continued with additional boxes in later sessions. Children, and even adults, may have a feeling of accomplishment as they look back over a cartoon story that has taken a number of sessions to illustrate. At termination of counseling, a book can be made of all the cartoon stories the client has created. Alternatively, this exercise may be used as a time line to encourage clients to talk about significant events in their life.

Here are some suggested therapeutic questions.

1. Looking back to the cartoons we made, was there anything you learned about yourself?

2. If you were to tell this story to your (biological/adoptive/foster) parents, what would you tell them? What would you *not* tell them?

3. How did you know this story would have this ending? What could you have done to make the ending different?

4. If you were to restart this story, where would you start?

5. Looking at the significant events in your life, which event has influenced/affected you the most? Tell me more about it.

6. If you were to add something or someone in this box [choose a significant piece], what and who would you add?

Fig. A3.1 How to fold the paper for the cartoon story

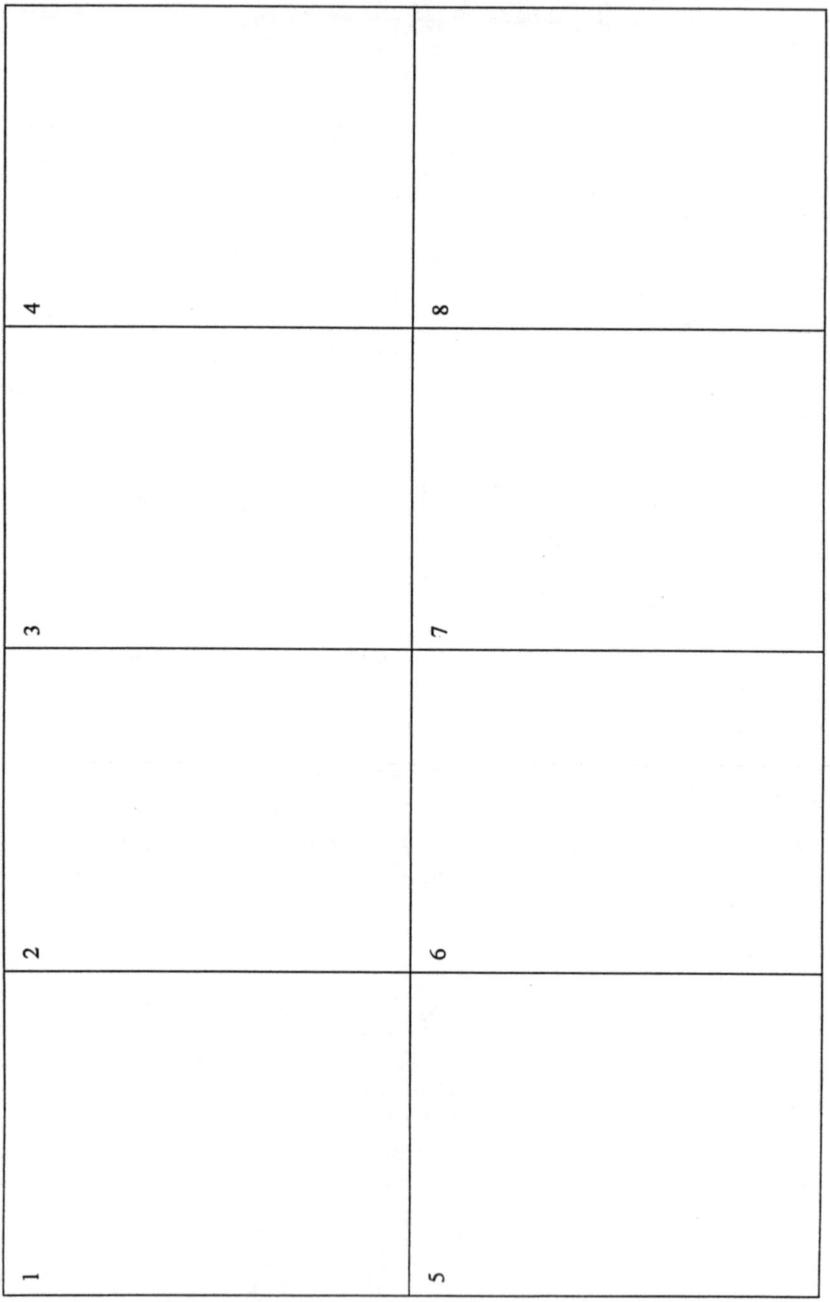

Deck of Feelings

Mark F. Akerlund

Items Needed

A deck of playing cards; glue or tape; scissors; feeling faces

Target Population

Children 5 to 11 who are inhibited, reserved, or guarded

Children who do not communicate or express feelings well

Purpose

To build rapport and assess client functioning

To increase clients' awareness of feelings and to gain understanding of how these feelings influence behaviors

To encourage expressions of feelings

Procedure

Before playing, copy the "feeling faces" sheet included in this book (fig. 3). Cut out each square, and glue or tape it on the back of a playing card.

You should participate in this game as a player. To begin, shuffle the cards and deal the deck to the players, making sure that all players have an equal number of cards.

Have the players select a card from their deck without looking, and place it number/face-side up in front of them. The player with the highest-value card wins all the cards turned over by the other players. In a tie, players with the highest cards each lay down another card. The winner collects the cards, chooses one of the feeling faces of these cards, and asks the player with the second-highest-value card, "What does this feeling mean to you?" or "Tell me about a time when you felt this way."

Continue the game until one player is out of cards. Game rules can be amended or modified to fit clients' needs.

Function in Assessment and Treatment

Assessment

Use this exercise to assist clients in exploring various feelings while increasing their awareness of what various feelings mean to them. You can also use it to ask clients about how different feelings influence their behaviors, and to encourage them to examine how other people experience the same feelings in similar and different ways.

Treatment

This game provides a bridge for processing complex feelings. For example, children can be asked to find a feeling from the collected cards that is associated with an experience of racism, discrimination, or cultural bias. If none of the cards seem to be appropriate to the child, he or she can create a new card. Therapeutically, you can suggest ways to communicate complex feelings. For example, "What could you say to someone who was treating you badly based on your race? How would you tell them this? What do you think this person's reaction would be? How would you handle their reaction and ensure your safety?"

A5
Don't Bug Me
Colleen Knox

Items Needed

Game board (see fig. A5.1); a die; a "bug" for each player (bug-shaped game piece, molded from Play-Doh or drawn and cut out); a set of Tell Me cards; a set of Feeling & Doing cards (table A5.1)

Target Population

Children 5 to 8 who have problems with anger control

Suitable for groups

Purpose

To help children understand that anger is an OK emotion when expressed appropriately

To help children think about how they handle their anger

To help children hear other options for handling anger

To encourage group cooperation

To help children think about other emotions and their reactions to them

Procedure

Have the child pick a bug game piece and place it on the Start square on the game board.

If used in groups, roll the die to see who goes first. Have players take turns in a clockwise order.

On each turn, the player rolls the die, moves the bug the number of spaces indicated, and follows the instructions on the space where the bug lands. He or she should draw a Tell Me card upon landing on the Tell Me space, and draw a Feeling & Doing card upon landing on the Feeling & Doing space. The events described on the Tell Me cards may or may not have been experienced by each child. If not, encourage the child to use imagination.

Whoever reaches or goes through the Happy Ending box will tell about a happy feeling.

Function in Assessment and Treatment

Assessment

This game is useful after an initial discussion about anger being an OK emotion and possible productive ways to handle anger. This game can help you assess whether the child is learning about anger, and whether he or she has developed constructive ways of handling it. This game also allows you to determine if other emotions need to be discussed.

Treatment

Through this exercise, children can begin to learn that feeling angry is OK, and that it can be expressed appropriately. They learn constructive ways of dealing with their anger through discussion with the therapist and one another. This game can be especially helpful for children who have difficulty identifying most or all of their feelings. Through discussion, they have the opportunity to learn what others feel in various situations.

Fig. A5.1 Game board for Don't Bug Me

START	Say one thing that's bugging you	Show your angry face	Show your sad face	TELL ME
FEELING & DOING	Move back 2 spaces	TELL ME	Say "Don't bug me!"	Make a happy face
Say "Ha, ha" 3 times	FEELING & DOING	How do you show someone that you like them?	Go forward 1 space	TELL ME
FEELING & DOING	TELL ME	Go forward 5 spaces	Relax!	TELL ME
TELL ME	Go forward 4 spaces	FEELING & DOING	Say one thing that's bugging you	Go back 2 spaces
TELL ME	Go back 3 spaces	TELL ME	Go forward 2 spaces	HAPPY ENDING

Table A5.1 Don't Bug Me cards

One side	The other side
TELL ME	Tell what you did and felt when a teacher yelled at you.
TELL ME	Tell what you did and felt when you found out you were going to go to Disney World.
TELL ME	Tell what you did and felt when your best friend told someone else one of your secrets.
TELL ME	Tell what you did and felt when your teacher said you cheated on a test, but you didn't.
TELL ME	Tell what you did and felt when you woke in the morning and were ready for school in ten minutes.
TELL ME	Tell what you did and felt when your teacher said, "Good job!"
TELL ME	Tell what you did and felt when you took something from someone without permission.
TELL ME	Tell what you did and felt when you found out your best friend was moving away.
TELL ME	Tell what you did and felt when your brother or sister was mean to you.
TELL ME	Tell what you did and felt when someone said something rude to you.
TELL ME	Tell what you did and felt when someone took your lunch money.
TELL ME	Tell what you did and felt when someone let the door close on you as you were about to walk through it.
TELL ME	Tell what you did and felt when a friend accused you of spreading rumors.
TELL ME	Tell what you did and felt when you found money in your pocket that wasn't yours.
TELL ME	Tell what you did and felt when you saw a friend being insulted or called names.
TELL ME	Tell what you did and felt when you yelled at someone you like.
TELL ME	Tell what you did and felt when you made good grades on your report card.

Table A5.1 (continued) **Don't Bug Me cards**

One side	The other side
FEELING & DOING	Show the face you make when you are angry.
FEELING & DOING	Tell one rule to follow when you are angry.
FEELING & DOING	Think about one thing that happened to you today that made you feel angry (or happy), then say loudly, "I am angry (or happy)!"
FEELING & DOING	What feelings do you have when you receive a gift? Say this feeling loudly.
FEELING & DOING	Show the face you make when you feel sad.
FEELING & DOING	What did you do the last time you felt angry?
FEELING & DOING	Pick a partner and show him or her how you would appropriately express your anger. Move forward 5 spaces!
FEELING & DOING	Pick a partner and show him or her how you would show you were happy. Move forward 5 spaces!
FEELING & DOING	What did you do the last time you felt happy?
FEELING & DOING	What is one good thing to do when you are angry?
FEELING & DOING	What do people do that makes you feel sad?
FEELING & DOING	When you are sad, what do you usually do?
FEELING & DOING	Is anger good or bad? How can you tell when it is good?
FEELING & DOING	Is anger good or bad? How can you tell when it is bad?
FEELING & DOING	When you are angry, what do you usually do?
FEELING & DOING	How do you feel when someone gives you a warm, friendly hug?
FEELING & DOING	Did you get angry today? What happened? How did you handle it?
FEELING & DOING	When were you happy today? What happened?

A6
Drawing a Person
Monit Cheung

Items Needed

Markers; pencil; "Drawing a Person" sheet (see fig. A6.1)

Target Population

Children or adults with communication issues

Purpose

To build rapport with the client

To help clients share their stories about communication or relationships, including parent-child relationship

To assess client functioning

Procedure

Give the "Drawing a Person" sheet (fig. A6.1) to the client and ask him or her to draw a person on the left side. Model the behavior.

Ask the client to draw another person on the right. Depending on the therapeutic purpose, this person can be anyone, of opposite gender to the first drawn person, a person different from the first drawn person, a person who likes (or dislikes) the first drawn person, or a friend or relative who listens to the first drawn person.

For rapport building, ask these questions after each drawing is done.

1. How old is this person?
2. Does she or he go to school? Does she or he have a job?
3. What is this person doing?
4. How many people are in his or her family?
5. What is the best/worst thing that has ever happened to him or her?
6. What makes this person happy? Sad? Mad? Laugh? Cry?
7. Does she or he have a friend?
8. What is this person's biggest worry? Biggest wish?

9. What does this person like best? What doesn't this person like?

10. What is his or her favorite TV show?

11. What changes would she or he like to see in the family?

12. Tell me more about this person.

For treatment, there are two options. For communication issues, ask the client to draw or write the preferred method to connect these two persons. Possible connection symbols include line, phone, conversational bubble, tree, house or common boundary, heart, and holding hands.

Ask questions to understand the client's preferred communication methods.

1. Tell me how these two people talk to each other.

2. Do they have anything in common?

3. What do they like to talk about?

4. If you were one of these people, what would you say to the other person to make this person understand you?

5. What does this connection method represent?

6. How would these two people improve their relationship?

7. What color/hobby/song does this person like?

8. What strengths/limitations does this person have?

9. If this "other person" were your father/mother (or a significant other), what relationship does this drawing show?

For relationship building, ask the client to draw a tree between these two persons. Don't suggest size, location, or type of tree because this tree may be presented as a barrier or enhancer to relationship building, depending on how it is drawn. Ask these questions.

1. Where is this tree located?

2. What's the one special thing about this tree?

3. What's the best/worst thing about this tree?

4. What kind of tree is this?

5. What are these two people doing?

6. How does each feel before and after the tree is drawn?

7. What's the one thing you would like to change about the tree?

8. Tell me more about this drawing.

9. If you would add something to this drawing, what would that be?

Function in Assessment and Treatment

Assessment

This game is adapted from the house-tree-person assessment in psychology (see Buck, 1970; Burns & Kaufman, 1970). In this exercise, you can facilitate reflections regarding self and self-image, and encourage clients to talk about connection and relationship between the two persons. This exercise also allows for free association, so that the client can relate thoughts to a significant person and image. For example, a female client who draws a man may share that her father no longer lives at home due to her parents' divorcing. Then she may draw the second person as her mother, and describe her as someone who provides for material needs but does not understand her emotional needs.

Treatment

Through expressive arts, you can identify clients' feelings associated with the descriptions of the drawing. Clients who are resistant to the idea of drawing a picture can choose different means of expressing themselves, such as writing (words or poems), coloring, or scribbling. The goal is to help clients gain a sense of release after sharing something about this significant individual in their life. In the house-tree-person game, clients can be encouraged to give a title to the drawing (or writing) that reflects its content and/or clients' feelings toward this drawing. This title can be changed or modified after clients share their views. The drawing and its title are both therapeutically empowering to clients in expressing themselves and are helpful in conflict resolution.

Fig. A6.1 Form for Drawing a Person

My name is _____ Age _____ Date of drawing _____ Therapist _____

Draw a person on this side.

The title of this drawing is _____

A7
Feeling Cubes
Lori Swan Provence

Items Needed

2 homemade cubes of the same size (e.g., 4" × 4" × 4"): On the sides of the person cube, write the name and draw a picture of mom, dad, sister, brother, uncle, or teacher (can be changed according to therapeutic purposes). On the sides of the feeling cube, write and draw feeling words (such as *happy, sad, excited, mad, calm, scared,* or other words from the feeling faces).

Target Population

Children 4 and up with issues related to feeling expressions

All cultures and socioeconomic backgrounds

Purpose

To break the ice

To build rapport

To encourage expressing feelings

Procedure

Ask the client to roll the two cubes (like dice) or to pick a person and a feeling from the cubes to discuss.

After an individual from the person cube and a feeling from the feeling cube have been selected, ask the client to describe something that this person has done (or might do) that would make him or her feel the specified feeling; for example, "Can you tell me about something that your uncle did that made him feel happy?" Alternatively, ask the client to think about something he or she has done (or might do) that would make the person feel that specified feeling; for example, "Think of something you could say that might make your mother angry."

The game may be repeated as many times as desired. The client can pass if he or she cannot think of an example or is not ready to discuss a particular subject. The client can also pass if something on one of the cubes does not apply to him or her, for example, if the client does not have a sister or brother.

The author of this game wishes to acknowledge Sandra K. Bruce for her helpful insights and suggestions.

Function in Assessment and Treatment

Assessment

This nonthreatening activity guides clients to begin expressing their feelings. It helps you begin to assess clients' recognition of and ability to express feelings, as well as to identify problems. Then use this game to help clients further explore and express their feelings, as well as to assess the problem(s) and begin to determine a potential plan of action.

Treatment

Use the cubes to help clients feel comfortable discussing a specific person or feeling, and to help clients explore how other people affect them and how they affect others. It can be used to help clients realize their problems or potential problems with regard to people and feelings, and to explore possible solutions to these problems.

1. Tell me how feelings can make you act in certain ways. Can the same feelings sometimes affect you in good ways/bad ways?
2. How do you know when a feeling is making you act in a certain way?
3. What do your parents/teachers do or say when they have a strong feeling toward someone or something?
4. What problems could you have if you expressed a feeling in an inappropriate way (not suitable to the occasion)?
5. What do you do or say to let people know how you feel? Is it appropriate? If not, how could express the feeling more appropriately?
6. When you dislike something in your family, what do you do or say? Let's (role-play) a situation with you and your mother/father/sister.

Feelings Hangman

Michele Ostrowski Taylor

Items Needed

Paper; blackboard or dry-erase board; chalk or markers; index cards

Target Population

School-age children who are able to read and write

Use caution with children who have experienced a violent trauma, as the hangman figure may be upsetting. Also, be aware that children who have recently immigrated to the United States may react negatively to the hangman because of their lack of previous exposure to this game. In these cases, use alternative figures instead (e.g., a circle-triangle-square figure, a house, etc.).

Purpose

To break the ice

To build rapport

To help clients express and name feelings they may experience

To educate clients about the coexistence of various feelings

Procedure

Make sure client understands how to play hangman.

1. Draw a hangman pole on the blackboard or dry-erase board (see fig. A8.1).

2. Ask the client to choose a feeling word for you (or the other person) to guess. (Use a feelings poster or cards to help the client choose words; e.g., feeling faces in fig. 3.)

3. Draw a line for each letter in the word. (Example: For the word *sad,* draw ____ ____ ____; see fig. A8.2.) Or use the lines provided in the example by adding or crossing out extras.

4. The other person (or the group) guesses letters that may be in the word, trying to guess the word.

5. Letters guessed correctly are placed on the appropriate line. Incorrect

guesses are written in a corner so that guessers can remember what they have said.

6. For each incorrect guess, the person who thought of the feeling word draws one part of a person on the hangman pole (e.g., the head, an arm, a foot).

7. The game is over when the word is guessed or when a complete person is drawn. Depending on the client, drawings can be very simple or get very detailed, adding things like hair, fingers, and clothes.

Take turns setting up the hangman game and guessing. Use only feeling words. Join in the game to show the client what is expected and to make it easier for him or her to participate.

At the end, write the word and encourage the clients to talk about this feeling. Explanations of what the feeling is like can be discussed, as can how one can tell if someone is feeling this way, ways to appropriately express this feeling, and examples of times when the client has felt this feeling or seen someone express this feeling.

In a group setting, one client can choose the word while the group tries to guess. The same discussions can occur, or the group can be asked to act out the feeling.

If a client (or group) is unable to think of a word, use index cards with feelings already written on them. Another option is to create these cards with clients before playing the game. With this method, the feeling words will apply to clients' current situation.

Function in Assessment and Treatment

Assessment

This game can be used to assess the ability of clients to conceptualize feelings and differentiate between various feelings. It can also be helpful for clients to identify feelings that they do not want to talk about or cannot express appropriately. While most clients show no particular reaction to the hangman figure, a reaction from the client could indicate experiences that should be explored.

Treatment

Used either individually or in a group, this game can help clients recognize feelings and understand that they can have mixed feelings at times. Ask clients probing questions during the game, for example, "Have you had this feeling recently? Tell me what happened."

Fig. A8.1 Form for Feelings Hangman

A B C D E F G H I J K L M

N O P Q R S T U V W X Y Z

Feeling Word

___ ___ ___ ___ ___ ___ ___ ___ ___

Fig. A8.2 Example of Feelings Hangman

Ⓐ B C Ⓓ E F G H I J K L Ⓜ

N O P Q R Ⓢ T U V W X Y Z

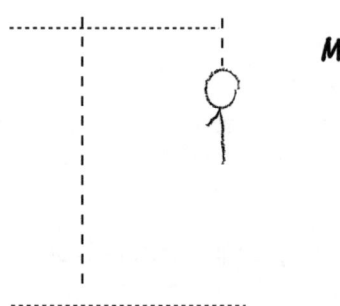

M

Feeling Word   S   A   D
              ___ ___ ___

Floating through Changes

Beth Tauber

Items Needed

Game board (see fig. A9.1); game pieces (blue, red, yellow, green); 4 colored pom-poms in a paper bag (blue, red, yellow, green); 4 crayons (blue, red, yellow, green); game cards (see table A9.1); 4 plastic eggs (blue, red, yellow, green); small prizes that can fit in the eggs

Target Population

Children (6 and up) and adolescents in foster care

Purpose

To assess functioning

To help abused and neglected children adjust and cope with transitions from moving from foster care back into their biological home or adoptive home placement

To facilitate discussion in a safe atmosphere regarding feelings about transitions in the child's life

Procedure

You and the client take turns decorating the spaces with the crayons (e.g., encourage players to draw items such as balloons or to color the entire square one color). Rotate colors equally.

Instruct each player to choose a game piece and to place it on the start position. To determine who will go first, each player picks one pom-pom from the bag. The individual who chooses blue will go first, then the order will be clockwise.

Have players put all the pom-poms back in the bag. Instruct the first player to take a pom-pom out of the bag, and then to move his or her game piece to the next space of that color. The player then takes a card of that color and follows the instruction on the card or answers the question.

After the game, each player will get the plastic egg that corresponds to his or her game-piece color. The plastic egg should have a prize inside.

Function in Assessment and Treatment

Assessment

This game can be used to assess the child's understanding of the transition of moving placements. It can also be used to assess any issues surrounding the change that are causing the child anxiety or stress. It is also helpful in assessing family functioning and support.

Treatment

This game enables children to express feelings about their family of origin, their foster/adoptive family, and themselves. It provides an atmosphere in which the child and family can openly share feelings. Use the game during visits with the foster/adoptive family and the family of origin. It should be used after rapport and trust have been developed.

This game can be modified for use with any population experiencing changes or transitions in their life (e.g., a child moving to a new school, a child newly diagnosed with an illness and returning home, terminating a therapeutic relationship, or letting go of a past event). Therapeutic questions should focus on the change and feelings related to adjusting to such change.

Fig. A9.1 Form for Changes

1 Start	2	3	4	5	6
12	11	10	9	8	7
13	14	15	16	17	18
24	23	22	21	20	19
25	26	27	28	29	30
36	35	34	33	32	31
37	38	39	40	41	42
48	47	46	45	44	43

Table A9.1 Game cards for Floating through Changes

Blue cards	Red cards
Move back 1 space.	What is your favorite cartoon show?
Skip a turn.	What is your least favorite cartoon show?
Move back 2 spaces.	
Switch places with the player in front of you.	Name your favorite cartoon character.
	What is your least favorite TV show?
Switch places with the player behind you.	What is your favorite movie?
	What do you like to do at home?
Move ahead 3 spaces.	What is your least favorite thing to do?
Take another turn.	If you could be doing anything right now, what would it be?
Move ahead 2 spaces.	
Move ahead 1 space.	What is your favorite story?
Draw another card of any color.	If you could meet anyone in the world, who would it be?
Draw another blue card.	
Move ahead 1 space.	If you could be anyone in the world, who would it be?
Move back to the last red space.	
Move ahead to the closest green space.	What would you like to study?
Move ahead to the closest yellow space.	What would you like to know about yourself?
	Who is your favorite person?
Move ahead to the closest red space.	Who would you like to be friends with?
Move back to the last blue space.	
Move ahead to the last blue space.	What is your favorite food?
Move back to the closest green space.	What is your favorite drink?
	What kind of fruit do you like?
Draw a green card.	

Table A9.1 (continued) **Game cards for Floating through Changes**

Yellow cards	Green cards
What animals remind you of your brothers and sisters?	I want my family to know that . . .
If you could have any animal as a pet, what would it be?	I am funniest when . . .
	I laugh when . . .
	If I had a magic potion, I would . . .
What animal reminds you of your foster mother?	When I am angry, I will . . .
What animal do you feel like today?	When I am happy, I will . . .
Flap your arms like a bird flying.	When I am sad, I will . . .
Stand on one leg like a flamingo.	When I am lonely, I will . . .
Moo like a cow 3 times.	If I could change one thing about myself, I would . . .
Gobble like a turkey 3 times.	My worst habit is/was . . .
Meow like a cat 3 times.	One thing I like to talk about is . . .
Make a fish face.	One thing I don't like to talk about is . . .
Bark like a dog 3 times.	One thing I will miss about my foster home is . . .
Hop like a bunny 3 times.	
Name a stuffed animal you have.	One thing I am looking forward to is . . .
What animal reminds you of your father?	One of my favorite things to do with my foster family is . . .
What animal reminds you of your mother?	A chore I do at home is . . .
	A chore I like to help with is . . .
What is your favorite animal?	A chore I don't like to do is . . .
If you could turn someone into a dog, who would this person be?	If I could change one thing about my family, it would be . . .
If you could turn your parent into an animal, what would it be?	

My "Family" Home

Kay Anderson and Laura G. Saunders

Items Needed

A toilet-paper or paper-towel tube; colored paper, contact paper, or gift wrap; 2–4 wide craft sticks; cotton balls (white or colored); yarn (for hair); 2 moveable eyes per cotton ball; glue; knife; scissors

Target Population

Children 5 to 12 in foster care

Purpose

To assess functioning

To provide a forum to discuss foster-home placements, reunification issues, children's return home, placement-home versus own-home placements, issues of divorce, step-families or blended families, family interactions (issues, roles, birth order)

To encourage expressing feelings

Procedure

Take the paper roll (use a paper-towel roll for families with more than three children) and cover it with any color paper, contact paper, or gift wrap. This "home" will be the out-of-home placement home or secondary home (divorce, foster care, step-, or blended family).

Make a second "home" that resembles the person's original home (biological family, or home where child resides most often in divorce, step-, or blended-family situations).

Use a sharp knife to cut two slots in the tube wide enough to insert the craft stick (see fig. A10.1A).

Take as many cotton balls (use colors to denote different people) as the number of parents or caretakers and decorate them with hair, moveable eyes, and faces (fig. A10.1B). Then glue the "parent" to the craft stick and insert it in the slot in the tube (fig. A10.1C). *Note:* If there are more than two caretakers in the home, glue two craft sticks end to end to include all adults in the home. Glue the sticks together after the first one is inserted into the slot.

Take as many cotton balls as there are children in the home and decorate them. Glue them to the second craft stick (figure A10.1D). *Note:* If there are more than three children, glue two wide craft sticks end to end to fit them.

Put the craft stick with the children inside the tube.

Ask the child to talk about the foster home or the secondary placement.

1. Who lives here?
2. What are the rules?
3. What are special things you do?
4. Are there special holidays?

Continue to explore how things are done in this home.

Ask the child to talk about how things are *different* when they go to visit their biological family (or other parent in a divorce situation).

1. Who lives in this house?
2. Are the rules different here?
3. Do you celebrate holidays the same?
4. How do you feel when you are in this home?
5. Are things different from when you lived here before?

Continue to explore the child's feeling, and the differences and similarities.

Vary the game by making the cotton balls into bunnies, pigs, ladybugs, or other creatures. Be creative and have fun!

Function in Assessment and Treatment

Assessment

Use this exercise to explore children's feelings about reintegration into their biological family's home, or to assess how children feel when visiting the "other parent" in a divorce situation or how they feel about step- or blended families.

Treatment

Use this activity to help the child discuss reunification with the biological parents so that the placement is successful. The child's feelings, fears, frustrations, and so forth can be discussed using the "homes." This activity is also useful to facilitate discussion on any other issue related to home placement.

Fig. A10.1 How to make my family home

A

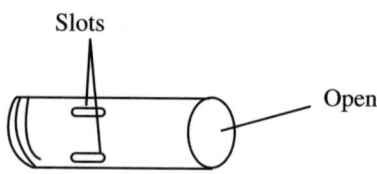

B

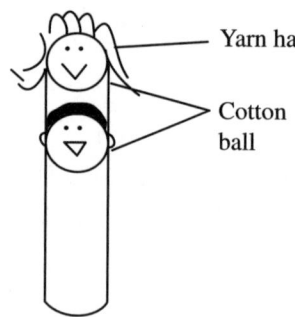

C

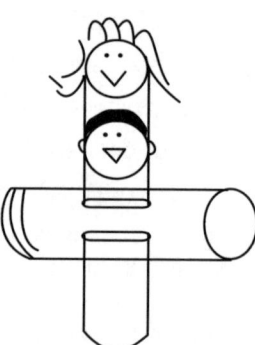

D

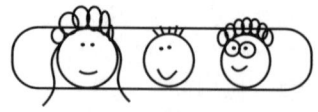

Glue 2 sticks here for 4 or more children

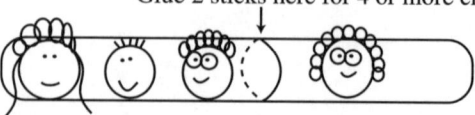

A11
My Friend's Story
Susan E. McCullough

Items Needed

A white vinyl tablecloth or a large piece of white fabric; crayons or colored markers; dolls or stuffed animals

Target Population

Children 3 to 8 in a therapeutic setting dealing with life or relationship issues

Individuals or groups discussing problem-solving skills

Purpose

To build rapport with the client

To assess the client's free-association skills

To identify the client's problems

To help the client develop problem-solving skills

Procedure

With the child, create a scene for the story. Ask the child to draw this scene. The scene could include houses, schools, parks, and so forth.

Ask the child to pick a "friend" from the dolls and stuffed animals.

Ask the child to tell a story about the selected friend. If a younger child has difficulty making up a story, ask the following questions:

1. What is this friend's name?
2. Is this friend a girl or a boy?
3. How old is this friend?
4. Is this friend sick or healthy?
5. Where does this friend live?
6. Who lives with this friend?
7. Does this friend go to school?
8. What does this friend like to do or play?

In a group, each child can answer a question or make up the next part of the story.

Function in Assessment and Treatment

Assessment

This activity can serve many purposes. Use it to help children feel more comfortable in the session, or to help identify and discuss children's problems, and allow children to use their imagination. You could use it as a first step to discussing a terminal illness with a young child, either his or her own or that of a family member. Observing the child in this exercise helps assess the child's developmental level. Don't read too much into the story; the child may be using her or his imagination, and is not necessarily projecting himself or herself into the story.

Treatment

This activity can help a child begin to resolve current life problems. For example, if a child does not want to go to school because the class bully teases the child, the story can be used to show the child new ways to deal with the problem. If the child is reluctant to discuss his or her terminal illness, this exercise can provide a nonthreatening avenue for expressing feelings, fears, and concerns. Similarly, if the child is unsure how to behave with a terminally ill family member, you can use the stuffed animal prop to help the child role-play appropriate responses.

A12
Operational Anger Release
Monit Cheung

Items Needed

Operation Skill Game by Milton Bradley; 2 D batteries; 25 3" × 2" pieces of index cards

Target Population

All ages, especially school-age children and adolescents

Children who have been sexually abused

Purpose

To help children recognize their right to protect their body

To help children release their feelings of anger or discomfort

To help children verbalize their feelings toward the abuse and the abuser

To assess a child's functioning

Procedure

Caution: Use this game therapeutically only after sexual abuse has been disclosed.

Place each of the plastic parts into its proper cavity in the "patient," and ask children about how to protect their body and why it is important.

Taking turns, have each player draw a Doctor card and then use the medical tweezers to remove the part indicated. After taking the part out (whether or not the child touches the edge), the player can use the tweezers to touch the edge of another cavity (of his or her choice) to cause the light and buzzer to activate.

Encourage each child to release anger and verbalize his or her feelings after the turn. Questions can be prewritten on a deck of index cards for the child to draw from, such as, "How do you feel?" "Say one thing to this 'patient' about your feeling." "What is it like to feel so helpless or defenseless?" "Make a facial expression to express your feelings."

After the game is over, debrief the child's feelings.

1. How did you feel when the "patient" was being touched by the tweezers?
2. What would you say to your abuser if he/she were here now?
3. What do you think about this game?
4. What insight does this game give to you?

Function in Assessment and Treatment

Assessment

Use this game for treatment after sexual abuse has been disclosed; it is not recommended as an assessment tool. It can help children release discomfort or anger associated with the abuse.

Treatment

The game itself is an anger-releasing device. During the game, ask questions about the child's feelings toward the abuse situation and the perpetrator. After the game, debriefing is recommended to allow the child to share more about how he or she thinks about this game and the abuse situation.

Sandy Feelings

Demori Currid Driver

Items Needed

Sand from a craft store; food coloring; sandwich bags; construction paper; glue; pencils, markers, or crayons; feeling faces (fig. 3); other art supplies if desired (e.g., beads, buttons, glitter, sequins, shells)

Target Population

Children 4 to 8 who have difficulty expressing feelings

Purpose

To break the ice

To encourage creativity

To encourage expressing feelings, especially difficult or complex feelings

Procedure

Pour approximately one cup of sand into a sandwich bag. Ask the child to select a food color, and add one or two drops. Do not add too much food coloring or the sand will become unworkable. Close the bag and allow the participant to shake and mix the bag until the food coloring is evenly distributed. Repeat for as many colors as desired. For a group, allow every child to mix a bag. Set the bags aside. Ask the child to think of an emotion, or discuss with the child an emotion that has been preselected as the theme of the session. Use the feeling faces as needed.

Ask the child to draw on a piece of construction paper a time when he or she felt this emotion. If the child cannot think of a time, brainstorm an imaginary situation where the child might feel this emotion. (If you want to discuss a particular situation that is relevant to the therapeutic process, i.e., visiting a sick relative, attending a new school, etc., simply assign the situation.) Allow the child to use any combination of pencils, markers, or crayons to complete the drawing. Provide feedback as the child is drawing, and engage the child in conversation about the elements of the picture.

Have the child outline all or part of the picture in glue. The child may also spread a thin layer of glue over an entire section. Allow the children to choose different colors of sand to sprinkle on the glue. Be sure to keep the picture flat as it dries, so that the glue will not run. Provide access to other available craft materials, such as beads, buttons, glitter, sequins, and shells.

Ask the children to discuss the elements in their pictures. Ask probing questions as necessary, for example, "How does it feel to be in that room you drew? The face in your picture is smiling; is that how you really feel?"

Function in Assessment and Treatment

Assessment

This activity allows children to express themselves creatively. The sand and art supplies engage children, and can promote a relaxed environment for them to discuss emotions and problems. Use the drawing as a basis for asking more detailed questions about the child's current situation.

Treatment

Use this activity at the beginning of a therapeutic session focusing on ways to cope with emotions and problems. If you selected the theme of fear, have the child draw a situation when he or she felt afraid, and then direct the rest of the session toward ways to control and handle fear. Upon termination of counseling, or when a sufficient number of drawings have been accumulated, combine all the drawings into a book and staple or bind them together. The child may decorate a cover for the book and title it "My Feelings Book."

A14

Somewhere over the Rainbow

Kristin Geiss-Curran

Items Needed

Drawing paper; 2 pens or pencils; crayons; feeling faces (optional; fig. 3)

Target Population

Children 6 and up and adolescents with emotional problem in school or at home

Brief counseling situations, such as in a school setting

Individuals or groups of 2

Purpose

To assess functioning

To help the client express feelings and identify coping strategies

Procedure

Listen to the client—do not minimize or exaggerate the child's feelings. Explain that all feelings are important, useful, and not to be labeled as good or bad.

This exercise may be adapted for a group of no more than four or six. Inform children that there are no right or wrong answers, and that what works for one person may not for another. You may want to prepare a worksheet containing blank stick figures, clouds, and rainbows to be filled in by the clients (fig. A14.1).

Present the child with a single piece of paper, and encourage him or her to construct a picture that tells a story of how she or he manages difficult emotions. Explain that the story should be organized into three parts: a storm cloud, a rainbow, and a fluffy cloud.

Ask the child to draw a person on the left side of the paper with the facial expressions that this person has whenever she or he is struggling with a problem. Over this person's head draw a storm cloud and write words in the cloud that describe how this person feels (e.g., sad, angry, lonely, etc.). Ask the child to imagine himself or herself in the person's situation. Encourage the child to tell the story based on the drawing.

Then compare it to a storm.

> "Even though the sun is still there, you can't see it because this big, thick cloud is blocking all its warmth, like sad feelings can sometimes block out our enjoyment of life" (or like scared or angry feelings can stop us from making friends, etc.).

> "Even though most of us like sunny days, the rainy days are very important too, just as it is important for you to let out sad feelings" (or angry feelings, scared feelings, etc.).

> "You can't control when the rain comes or how long it lasts, just like you can't control many of the things that happened to you" (or when our sad feelings come, etc.).

After thoroughly exploring what the child sees as his or her "storm cloud" feelings, continue the story by asking what sometimes appears when the rain stops and the sun starts to shine through the remaining clouds (a beautiful rainbow). Draw a rainbow connecting the storm cloud to a new cloud on the right side of the page (see fig. A14.1). Leave spaces between the lines of the rainbow for the child to write things she or he can do to feel better. You can write for young children.

Draw a white, fluffy, marshmallow cloud. Ask the child to draw a picture of how she or he would like to feel beneath a cloud. Write words that describe the child's desired feelings (e.g., happy, loved, safe, etc.) inside the cloud.

Ask the child to imagine doing the things written in the rainbow in order to slide over to the soft, fluffy cloud. Tell the child to use the story picture as a reminder of what to do when things in life are stormy.

Function in Assessment and Treatment

Assessment

This activity helps assess how well the child deals with powerful emotions, as well as what tools the child already uses and can build upon. It also helps build rapport and provides a foundation for discussing other issues that emerge. See examples in figure A14.2 and A14.3.

Treatment

This activity helps children express feelings, and it provides an opportunity to teach and reinforce that all emotions are important. It can open discussion about what is within the child's control and what is not, which can be an important teaching tool. It helps clients realize that no matter what their situation, they can still make some choices. It also empowers clients to recognize that they possess the ability to find coping strategies or to seek help when they need it.

Fig. A14.1 Form for Somewhere over the Rainbow

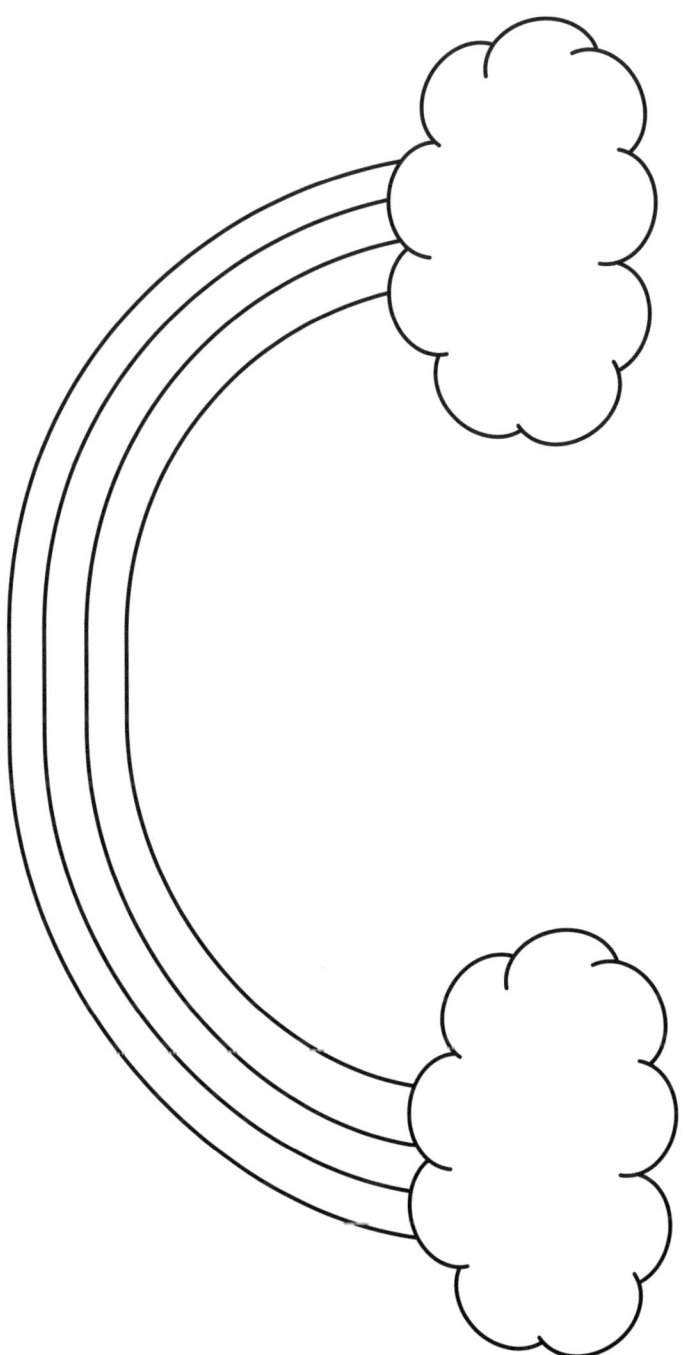

Fig. A14.2 Sample drawing for Somewhere over the Rainbow, drawn by an eight-year-old girl who had been sexually abused

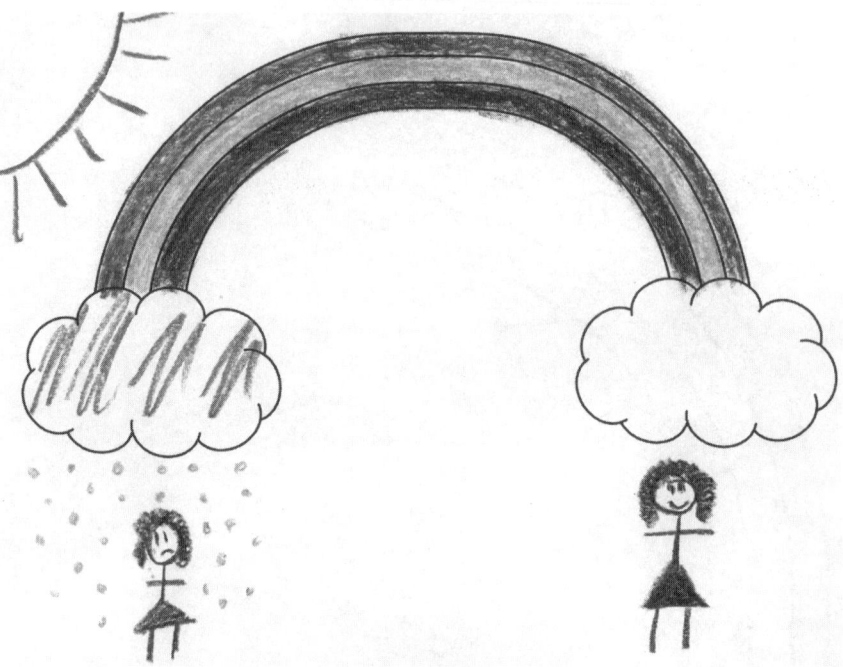

Fig. A14.3 Sample drawing for Somewhere over the Rainbow, drawn by an eight-year-old boy who was disruptive in class

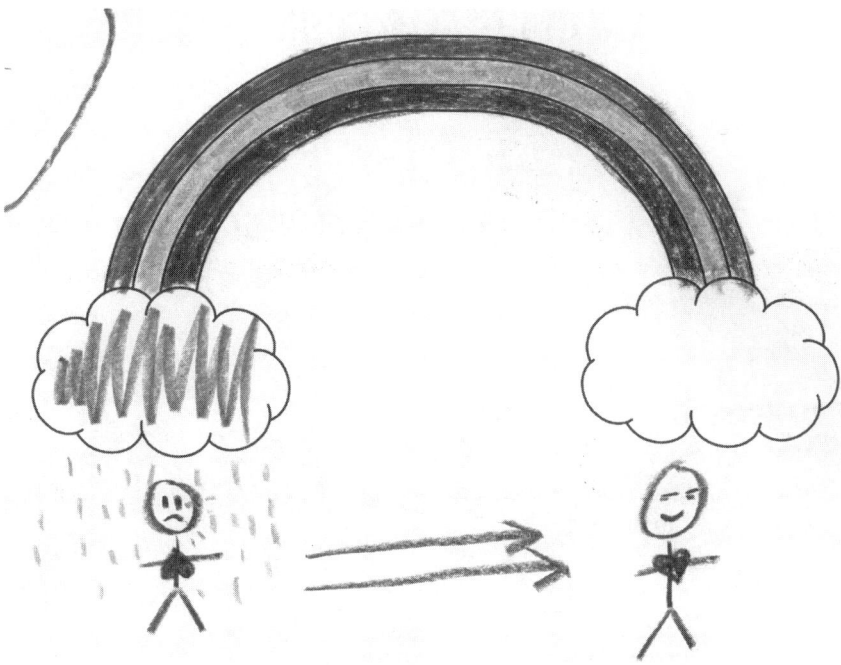

A15
This Is My Friend
Wing-sai Dion Or

Items Needed

Plastic egg(s); markers; "Our Shared Moments" sheet (fig. A15.2)

Target Population

Children 5 to 15 who bully others

Purpose

To build rapport

To assess social relationships and social needs, noting quality of social and emotional interactions

To help clients develop empathy

To introduce positive peer relationship to clients

To help clients acknowledge the consequences to themselves of their behavior

To help clients acknowledge the consequences to others of their behavior

Procedure

Begin by presenting a decorated egg to the child as "my best friend" (see fig. A15.1). Explain to the child that he or she will decorate an egg in a similar way, and provide markers and eggs.

Allow 3–6 minutes to decorate the egg with a face. Have the child print "my best friend" on the egg. The egg can be designated as male or female.

Instruct the child to create a name for this new "friend" and to introduce him or her.

Discuss how to share time with and care for this new friend. Provide the child with the sheet "Our Shared Moments" (fig. A15.2).

Allow the child time to do the activities with this friend, and instruct him or her to record activities on the "Our Shared Moments" sheet. The child should be allowed to take the friend home.

Children may not follow instructions to care for the egg. Use positive reinforcement to encourage appropriate participation.

Emphasize the following guidelines:

1. Take care of the friend's safety (no broken eggs!).
2. Engage in the brainstormed activities with the friend.
3. Record activities.
4. No cheating (i.e., no replacing a broken egg).
5. No neglecting the egg.

The child brings the friend to the next session for debriefing.

Function in Assessment and Treatment

Assessment

This exercise helps build rapport and encourages positive interaction. It also connects sessions to increase commitment to the therapy. Through drawing and introduction, projection can be observed. The clinician can also analyze the brainstormed activities in order to make initial assessments on the peer relationships and social needs.

Treatment

By caring for the egg's safety during the week, the child develops empathy, caregiving skills, and a sense of responsibility. The debriefing session serves as a forum for a discussion on bullying, and can help the child acknowledge behaviors. The exercise can also serve as a means to discuss positive peer relationship. In using the egg, anxiety and defense mechanisms associated with disclosing bullying behavior can be deflected.

Fig. A15.1 My friend the egg

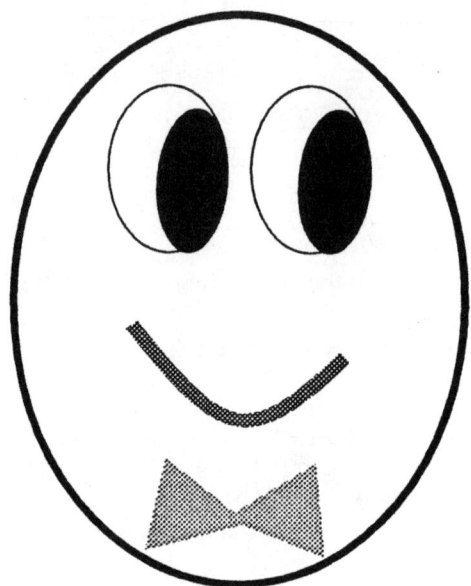

Fig. A15.2 Diary of shared moments

Our Shared Moments!!

Name _____

	SUN	MON	TUE	WED	THU	FRI	SAT
Sunshine							
Shower							
Chat							
Give it to someone							
Accident ☹							
Others							

A16

When I Feel . . .

Othea G. McCoy-Clinton

Items Needed

8 feelings/emotions cards; color-coded board with a spin dial in the middle; 2 dice

Target Population

Children 7 and up and adolescents with emotion-related problems

All socioeconomic backgrounds

Purpose

To assess functioning

To encourage expressing feelings

Procedure

Prepare a game board with a spin dial in the middle and color-coded sections representing various emotions (orange = happy; yellow = excited; pink = calm; black = uncertain; red = angry; brown = lonely; blue = sad; white = any feeling). See figure A16.1.

Prepare feelings/emotions cards. The cards should designate the same eight emotions as the game board and have the same colors as above. Write the emotion on the card. Draw or glue a picture of a facial expression corresponding to the emotion on the same side. Place these cards face-down in the eight sections on the game board, but take care not to block the spin dial.

In groups, players throw the dice to determine who goes first. The player with the lowest number spins first, and the others will follow in a clockwise order. After each spin, the player pulls the card from the section the dial points to. The player states the emotion on the card and then completes the sentence, "I feel _____ when . . ." by describing an actual situation or occasion that provoked that feeling.

Encourage the sharing of experiences (e.g., Close your eyes and think of this emotion; what did you see? Give a word that is related to this emotion. Identify a situation that can make you feel this emotion.). Conclude the game when the last emotion card has been revealed and shared.

Function in Assessment and Treatment

Assessment

This exercise can help assess emotional issues and mixed feelings. It is also a means to help children or adults develop and strengthen communication skills while rebuilding self-esteem. It can be used to engage a nonverbal child. You could also use this exercise to identify inappropriate behaviors or responses.

Treatment

Engage clients by asking them to comment on their feelings/behaviors, or to identify alternative responses/behaviors when dealing with certain emotions and feelings (e.g., What else could you have done? Can you share another time when you were happy? That sounds scary; what did you do?).

Fig. A16.1 Game board for When I Feel . . .

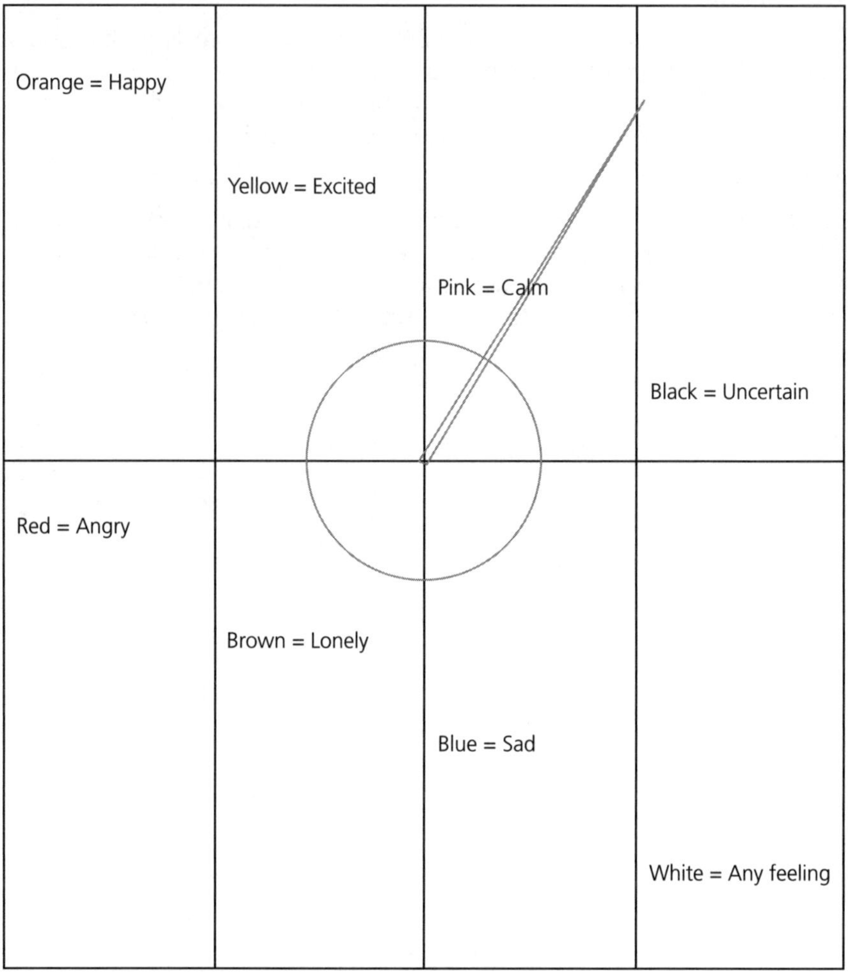

Orange = Happy

Yellow = Excited

Pink = Calm

Black = Uncertain

Red = Angry

Brown = Lonely

Blue = Sad

White = Any feeling

Therapeutic Games and Activities for Families and Groups

Bag It!

Robin Doak Neyrey

Items Needed

Brown-paper lunch bags; index cards; markers or crayons; self-stick notes (3" × 3"); feeling faces (fig. 3)

Target Population

Children or adults who feel disempowered

Purpose

To break the ice

To build rapport

To encourage expressing feelings

To enhance self-image

To provide cognitive restructuring/empowerment

Procedure

Feeling Identification and Exploration

Ask clients to decorate a bag with an image of themselves or something that represents them, such as colors, shapes, and favorite items.

Ask clients to identify three to five feelings they have experienced in the past week or month that require their immediate attention, and write each feeling on a self-stick note. They may use a chart of feeling faces for assistance.

Instruct clients to consider whether they are comfortable sharing these feelings with others. Clients should place the notes containing feelings they are comfortable expressing on the outside of the bag, and the notes containing feelings that they prefer to keep to themselves on the inside of the bag.

Review the choices and explore the placement of feelings with clients. Ask probing questions to explore patterns, the feelings induced by the exercise, any new awareness or understandings, and so forth.

Affirmations

Decorate a bag using the same procedure as above.

Ask clients to write affirmations on index cards and place them in the bag for daily use. Examples: "I am a good person," "I am lovable," "I am precious," "I am able to manage my emotions," "I can make good decisions," "I can feel my feelings without judging myself."

Card readings may be assigned as a daily exercise or for personal use as daily or periodic support.

Cognitive Restructuring/Empowerment

Decorate a bag using the same procedure as above.

Ask clients to write cognitive restructuring statements on index cards that reflect the area of therapeutic concern. Examples: "I can manage my anger," "I am able to think before I respond," "I can show my angry feelings without losing control," "I can relax," "I am able to express my anger feelings appropriately," "I am responsible for my own behavior."

Card readings may be assigned as a daily exercise or for personal use as daily or periodic support.

Function in Assessment and Treatment

Assessment

Use these exercises to assess clients' self-image, identify clients' feelings, encourage the expression of feelings, and maximize attention span, creativity, and verbal and motor skills.

Treatment

The feeling identification and exploration exercise provides an opportunity for educating clients regarding the wide range of possible emotions. It can increase clients' awareness of behavior patterns and verbal expressions associated with behavior. The sharing process encourages an understanding of the universality of human emotions, and allows clients to experience interpersonal connectedness. The affirmations and cognitive restructuring exercises help clients learn alternative cognitive techniques and rehearse the new learning. The affirmation exercise is useful for all levels of clinical intervention, aiming at enhancing self-image through positive self talk.

A18

Childhood Memories

Monit Cheung

Items Needed

Sheet of paper; pens and colored markers

Target Population

All ages, especially adolescents or adult survivors of childhood traumas

Purpose

To assess functioning

To encourage clients to recall some childhood memories for processing feelings

To psychoanalyze remembered situations

To discuss the positive images of childhood events

Procedure

Ask the clients to write down three concrete objects that can be related to childhood memories. The clients do not need to go into details of how these items relate to the memories. Give suggestions only if the clients cannot think of anything (e.g., a toy, a pillowcase, a photo, a drawing, a dress, a coat, a report card).

As a homework assignment, ask the clients to bring these items to the next session. If the items no longer exist or cannot be located, instruct the clients to bring any other childhood item or something to serve as a substitute. For example, have the clients bring a used pillowcase instead of a treasured childhood pillowcase, or a new stuffed toy instead of the stuffed toy from their childhood.

In the next session, ask the clients to concentrate their thoughts on one item at a time while answering the following questions:

1. What are your reasons for including this item on the list?

2. What was the significant meaning of this item in your childhood?

3. What is the significant meaning of this item to you *now*?

4. What insight can you gain from this item at this moment?

Function in Assessment and Treatment

Assessment

Many clients do not keep childhood items, and this exercise can help them talk about childhood memories and their impact. Items from childhood can help clients uncover repressed memories. If a client continually forgets to bring any items, it may be time to address repression of memories. Explain the importance of letting pleasant memories as well as unpleasant ones surface in order to achieve therapeutic goals. Use this exercise also to encourage the client to recall happy memories, no matter how insignificant the item seemed to be.

Treatment

This exercise takes place in two sessions: (1) discuss the function of memories; (2) identify the influence of one's upbringing in one's current situation. The items can help clients realize that repression is often used as a defense mechanism to deal with stress and anxiety. Even if the items were not brought in, you should encourage clients to talk about the items as they are related to both their childhood and current situations.

A19
Chinese Adoption
Kit-ying Anny Ma

Items Needed

A plastic egg for each child (or doll or a simple paper drawing of a human figure); sheets of paper (8½" × 11"); colored pens or markers; at least 20 keys cut from paper (i.e., paper in a key shape); stickers

Target Population

Chinese children 5 to 11 adopted by American couples

Purpose

To build rapport

To assess whether American couples should talk about adoption issues with their adopted Chinese children

To allow adopted Chinese children to recognize that incorporating both American and Chinese identity is advantageous

To encourage expressing feelings surrounding adoption

Procedure

Ask the adopted Chinese children to decorate their plastic egg with the stickers, pens, and markers to make it a "baby." (The race of the baby should be the same as that of the children's adopted parents.)

Invite the children to pretend to be a parent caring for the baby, and ask them what they would do, such as feeding or teaching the baby. Assess the children's experiences of taking care of the baby to ascertain whether they seem to be open to adopting a baby of a different race.

If the timing is right, ask the children about the meaning of adoption; if not, continue the game by exploring the strengths of incorporating both an American and a Chinese identity.

Ask the children to draw a symbol to represent them at the center of a piece of paper. Prompt the children to write down or draw the most significant problems they are faced with, especially related to identity and racial issues, around the symbol they drew.

Discuss the strengths of having an American identity. When children express a strength, prompt them to draw a circle representing a protective shield against the difficulties that surround the symbol of the self. Also provide the children with a paper key (i.e., solution to their problems) when they think of a strength. Children may color the shield and the key in a favorite color.

Discuss the strengths of having a Chinese identity with the children. Prompt the children to draw an additional protective shield, and provide an additional paper key. The new shield layer and key might be colored with a different color.

Continue the game until five to ten strengths are found. Ask the children how they feel about having two racial identities.

Function in Assessment and Treatment

Assessment

The activity assesses whether the timing is appropriate for couples to discuss adoption issues with their adopted Chinese children. If the children talk about adoption when creating the "baby," you can prepare the parents to tell their children about the adoption process in the next session. You can also use the game to assess children's ability to understand their cultural heritage and strengths.

Treatment

Through this game, children will be empowered to acknowledge their strengths related to their racial identities. Children can learn that they do not need to choose either American or Chinese identity, because incorporating both identities can protect them from certain adversities and enhance resilience as they face racial problems.

A20
Clay Therapy
Monit Cheung

Items Needed

Several cans of Play-Doh, or homemade clay; plastic placemat or transparent plastic with white paper under it; digital camera (optional)

Clay ingredients: 2 cups flour; 1 cup salt; 4 teaspoons cream of tartar, 2 packages unsweetened Kool-Aid; 2 cups water; food coloring (optional); 2 tablespoons vegetable oil. See Bishop 2005 for more homemade recipes.

Target Population

Children 6 and up, adolescents, or adults

Very young children or nonverbal children

All cultures and socioeconomic backgrounds

Purpose

To break the ice

To build rapport

To assess developmental stage, capabilities, motor skills, strengths, and problems

To clarify problem definition

To develop a treatment plan

To intervene therapeutically

Procedure

Get several cans (assorted colors) of Play-Doh, or use this recipe. Measure and mix flour, salt, cream of tartar, and Kool-Aid in a large bowl. Add 2 cups of boiling water to the dry ingredients and mix them. Add several drops of food coloring for a more vivid color. Add vegetable oil and mix well.

Knead the mixture together until it is very well mixed and has the consistency of clay dough. If too wet, use medium heat and stir the mixture constantly for 1–2 minutes or until the dough thickens. Allow mixture to cool. Store clay in a covered plastic container in the refrigerator when not in use.

Instruct each client to use a plastic placemat (or transparent plastic with a piece of white paper underneath) and to create a clay figure on it. Depending on the theme, ask each participant to create something that comes to his or her mind. *Note:* Snakes and round balls are common; don't overreact to clients' creations.

Ask each participant to explain what he or she has made, or to use each creation to tell a story.

Take a digital photo of each creation or save the entire creation for the next session. In following sessions, clients can add new creations to identify feelings, fears, or concerns.

Function in Assessment and Treatment

Assessment

Clay modelling can be used to assess fine motor skills while helping clients release unwanted anxiety and tension. By examining the client's creation, the therapist can assess the client's perception of the presenting problem by asking questions such as,

1. What is this?
2. What does this color represent?
3. How does this creation help you resolve your concern/fear/problem?
4. How did you feel when you played with the clay?
5. Does this creation remind you of your concern/fear/problem?

Treatment

Use the creation to address the client's concern. Ask each client to think of a solution based on what she or he made. By examining the creations, you can facilitate a discussion about the client's situation and its solution. The colors and shapes can stimulate the client's thinking to find his or her own solutions.

Color-Code Chronology
Laura G. Saunders

Items Needed

Color-code charts (see figs. A21.1, A21.2); paper (8½" × 11" or larger); box of crayons or markers

Target Population

Children or adults

Groups

Purpose

To enhance awareness of feelings

To encourage discussion of past and current life events

To assess clients in a nonthreatening manner

Procedure

Have clients complete the Color Code of Feelings (fig. A21.1). Clients should consider what emotions are represented by the colors, and write a particular feeling next to each color listed. Alternatively, give clients feeling words to associate with colors (fig. A21.2). *Note:* When selecting feeling words for figure A21.2, you and/or the clients can choose words that are significant to the clients' current life situation.

After completing a code page, discuss clients' responses.

Using a blank sheet of paper, have clients draw a time line from their birth to the present. Instruct clients to select significant life events to note on this time line.

Have clients refer to their color code. Tell them to use the colors to represent their feelings during specific life events, and to mark the colors on the time line in the appropriate time frame. Clients may divide time by groups of years, by developmental periods (early childhood, middle childhood, adolescence, etc.), or in any other meaningful way. The amount of color used should be in direct proportion to the amount of the specific feeling the client recalls having during that time (i.e., if yellow signifies happy, and during a specific time the client was happy about three-fourths of the time, then three-fourths of that time period should be filled in with yellow). See figure A21.3.

Be sure to focus on the process, not the end product. After the time line chart is completed, discuss the feelings and their association with the life events listed on the time line. Some areas to discuss are negative feelings, positive feelings, how the time line was divided, and perceptions of significant life events by different family or group members.

Function in Assessment and Treatment

Assessment

Use the color code as an assessment tool to identify clients' feelings, especially mixed feelings during a particular time in their lives. It is therapeutically helpful for those who have not expressed emotions for a long time to encourage them to visualize the change of feelings after the occurrence of a family crisis or a significant event.

Treatment

Identify to clients that feelings can be positive or negative. Within the same family, each member may perceive change in a different way and therefore feel differently than others. With this in mind, clients can move forward to generating a new set of feelings and expectations toward the foreseeable future.

Fig. A21.1 Key for color code of feelings: colors

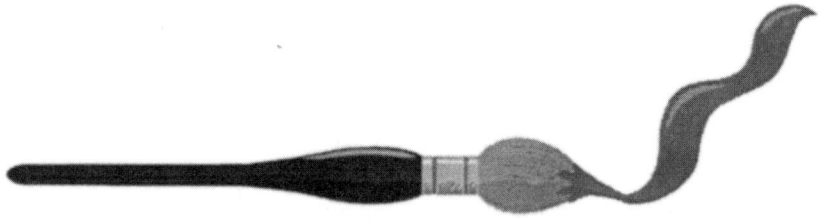

COLOR CODE OF FEELINGS

Red _____

Blue _____

Yellow _____

Green _____

Purple _____

Black _____

Brown _____

Gray _____

Orange _____

Other color _____

Name _____   Date _____

Fig. A21.2 Key for color code of feelings: feelings

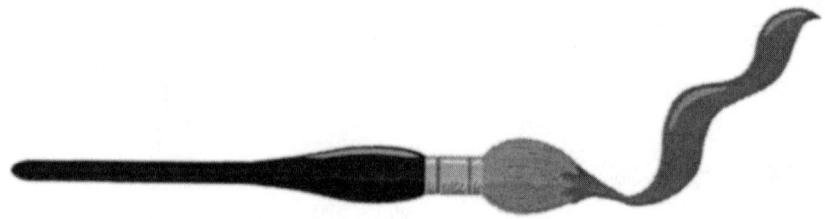

COLOR CODE OF FEELINGS

Happy _____

Sad _____

Angry_____

Lonely _____

Love _____

Scared _____

Frustrated _____

Jealous _____

Rage _____

Grief _____

Satisfied _____

Guilty_____

Other feeling _____

Name _____   Date _____

Fig. A21.3 Sample color-code time line

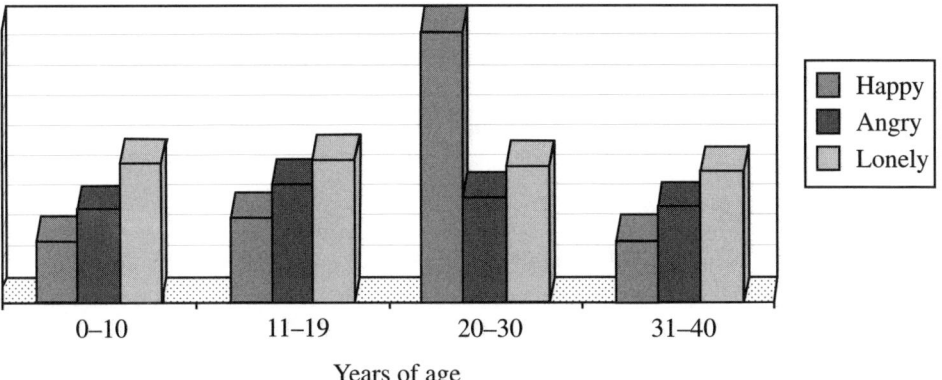

A22
Colorful Expressions
Laila Amir Narsi

Items Needed

White paper (2" × 3"); colored paper (8½" × 11"); crayons, markers, or color pencils; tape; glue; small beads or other small items; a basket

Target Population

Children, adolescents, or adults exploring self-awareness

Purpose

To break the ice

To help clients construct and express positive feelings for other family or group members

To promote group cohesiveness and communication

To increase feelings of self-awareness and self-worth

Procedure

Ask participants to sit in a circle. Have them write their name on a small piece of white paper, fold it up, and put it in a basket.

Ask each participant to choose a sheet of colored paper.

Pass the basket around the circle so each participant can pick a name. If someone selects his or her own name, he or she should put the paper back in the basket and try again.

Have each member write the selected name in large letters on the sheet of colored paper. They can use the markers, beads, and so forth to decorate the name as they like, in two minutes. Then they should choose one positive word describing this person and decoratively display this word on the paper. Encourage members to write only positive words. If participants can't think of positive words, they should pass.

Pass the paper around to each group member, who will have one minute to decoratively add a different positive word to describe this person. Each group member may use any of the art supplies.

After everyone has had a turn to add a positive word to all the names, debrief with the clients. Use the following sample statements:

1. Read and discuss the words on your sheet.

2. Which is your favorite word, and why?

3. How does it feel to write these positive words and decorate the sheet?

4. How does it feel to receive these positive words and a decorated sheet?

5. How would you feel if no one could think of positive words to describe you?

6. How does it feel to be able to design this sheet in your own way?

7. Would you like to use art in your future activities?

Function in Assessment and Treatment

Assessment

Use this exercise to assess clients' ability to positively describe another family or group member and therefore increase self-esteem. This game builds rapport and enhances group communication while allowing clients to exercise their imagination. It helps identify family or group members who are uncomfortable with complimenting another member or themselves. If participants use negative or cruel words, help the group process their feelings and discuss why words can hurt.

Treatment

Often, giving compliments to another person can be difficult, even when positive aspects of a person are known. This activity promotes the expression of positive feelings toward others. It enables clients to encounter descriptions of themselves and others that they may not have realized earlier. Use this activity to encourage open communication, and to improve group cohesiveness and self-esteem.

A23
Connections
Heather Alden Pope

Items Needed

Fabric sack (pillowcase); card-stock game board divided into four quadrants and labeled with four words describing a value or theme to stimulate discussion (e.g., fig. A23.1); 12–16 items that symbolically represent the game-board themes (e.g., key, doll, chore chart, whistle, small heart, candle, plastic spoon taped on a paper plate, small mask, framed picture, stop sign, toy phone, happy face, angry face; see fig. A23.2)

Target Population

Children, adolescents, or adults—can be modified for use with all age levels

Families, parent-child dyads, small group sessions

All cultures and socioeconomic backgrounds

Purpose

To break the ice

To build rapport and stimulate discussion

To assess functioning

Procedure

Prior to beginning the game, make sure that the players understand each word on the game board. Prompt players to demonstrate their understanding by asking them to give an example of each term. For example, "Rituals & Celebration" can be a holiday celebration, a birthday party, a reunion dinner, or a religious ceremony. Ask questions such as "When was the last time you had a celebration or ritual?"

Present the game board, and explain that each player will have the opportunity to draw objects out of the sack and place them on the board next to the word that symbolically represents that object. Explain that there is no limit to the number of items that can be placed on each word, and there are several possible outcomes.

Prompt the player to draw the objects out of the sack one by one until all of the objects have been placed on the board. Ask the player to choose a quadrant and share why he or she placed each item in that square. Ask the player probing questions such as, "How does this item connect with this word?" Encourage the player to make connections between the objects and the other words on the game board.

Give each player a turn to make and describe their choices. The game can continue as long as it facilitates discussion. The game may continue in a following session by having clients bring in new items for the sack. Or you could place the objects on the board and have clients describe them.

Function in Assessment and Treatment

Assessment

This game is intended to stimulate discussion with clients and facilitate your growing relationship with the clients. Through active listening, you can get a sense of how clients interpret the world. You may discover that what you perceived as an object for one quadrant was interpreted differently by a client, based upon divergent thought processes and life experiences.

When a small group play the game, each player takes a turn drawing an object out of the sack and placing it on the game board. In small groups, some players may think that an object was placed in the wrong quadrant. In such cases, remind the group that the purpose of this game is to make connections, and all of the possible solutions will be discussed when the sack is empty.

With families or parent-child dyads, the child(ren) may place the objects first and share their connections, and then the parent(s) may move some of the objects around and share their connections. These rearrangements may stimulate communication on how one's perceptions can be different for the same objects and may encourage each individual to try to "see" from the other's point of view.

Treatment

Assess clients both while they are deciding where to place the objects and during discussion of the connections. Ask the clients about the thought processes in placing each object. You should also challenge the clients to see any other possible connections. You might choose to self-disclose where you would have placed an object and why. This is an effective way to build rapport and stimulate conversation.

This game can reveal some areas of a client's life that may warrant discussion in future sessions. For example, if the client places the paper plate and plastic spoon on Rituals & Celebration and relates that his family frequently has picnics together, you might explore other family rituals, such as religious or spiritual events. If the client places the plate and spoon on Responsibility and says that she understands that eating is a responsibility since recovering from an eating disorder, you might explore eating disorders and patterns of eating.

Modifications include using pictures instead of words on the game board for younger children, clients with special needs, or clients with limited English proficiency. Different words and objects could be used, depending upon the clients and their situation.

Fig. A23.1 Sample game board for Connections

Responsibility	Relationships
Rituals & Celebration	Safety

Fig. A23.2 Sample symbols for Connections

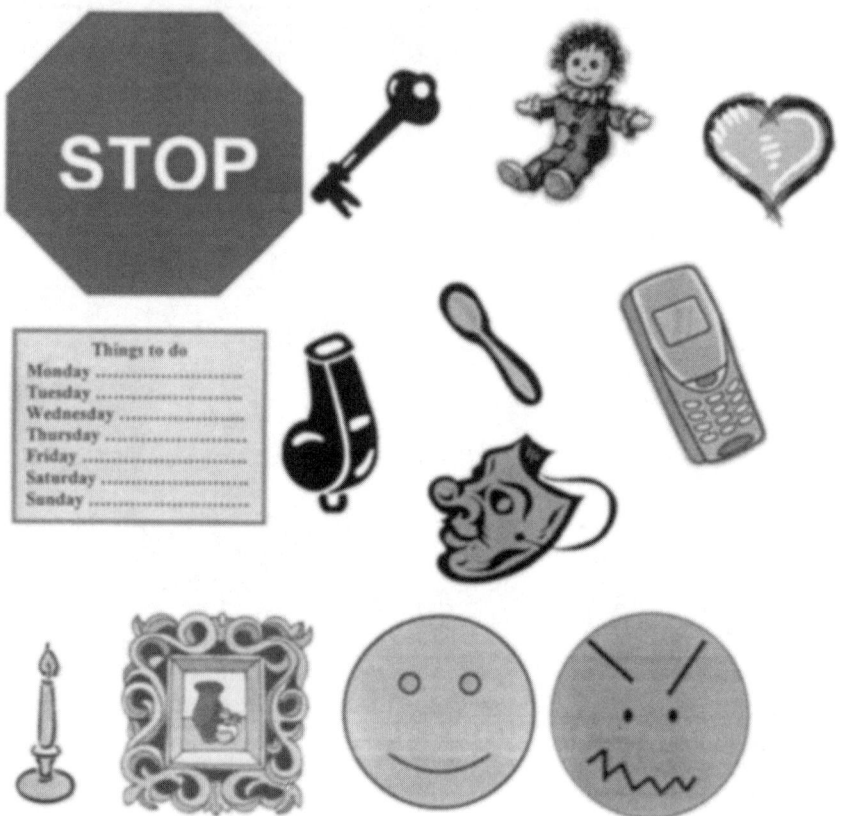

A24

Designing a Board Game

Monit Cheung

Items Needed

Game board, (fig. A24.1 for groups, A24.3 for individuals); colored markers; tokens; game pieces; 2 dice

Target Population

Clients of all ages

Groups, families, or individuals

Purpose

To break the ice

To build rapport/relationships

To promote cooperation among family or group members

To assess family and group dynamics

Procedure

Group Activity

Arrange groups of two or three clients. Copy the game-board sheet (fig. A24.1), and explain to the groups that they will be designing a game.

Set up a theme for therapeutic purposes (e.g., building relationships, how to become happier, family communication). Within the parameters of the therapeutic theme, the game should have the following components: (1) title, (2) purpose, (3) rules and procedures, and (4) the "Design Our Board Game" sheet (fig. A24.2).

Encourage group members to be creative. They should take approximately fifteen minutes to design the game. The group will play the game and modify the procedures, if necessary, before presenting it to the entire group.

Prompt each small group to demonstrate how to play the game and how it fits the theme. Facilitate discussion of each game.

Individual Session

Set a theme for the game based on the client's current situation.

Throw the die first and move your game piece on the game board provided (fig. A24.3). On an empty space, write, draw, or color something related to the theme. Instruct the client to do the same.

Ask the client about his or her writing or drawing.

1. What does the word _____ mean?
2. What does _____ [color] represent?
3. You wrote here that you are not happy; what would you (or your significant other) do to make you feel happier?

On a space that has already been decorated, the player should comment about the content of the space.

If the client does not want to write or draw, she or he can make a comment or facial expression, which you can write or draw for the client.

End the game at any time or when the client seems ready to discuss something revealed during the game.

Function in Assessment and Treatment

Assessment

In an individual session, use this activity to assess client problems when clients do not wish to disclose information or feelings. Model participation to encourage clients to get involved. Once some key words or feelings are revealed in the activity, ask the client to elaborate by saying, "Tell me more about it" or "How does this relate to our theme?" In a family or group session, this activity encourages each member to participate in decision making, so that you can identify each member's strengths and weaknesses in dealing with family or group dynamics.

Treatment

This is a solution-focused treatment tool for individual, family, or group settings. When the family or group members design an activity for themselves in a relaxed manner, they tend to use their full potential to identify and resolve issues. The completed game board can be used for future therapeutic analysis. Although you could use this game to compare the past and the present, such analysis should primarily focus on how clients perceived their writing or drawing at the time of therapy, and what directions they would like to take to resolve their problem.

Fig. A24.1 Blank game board

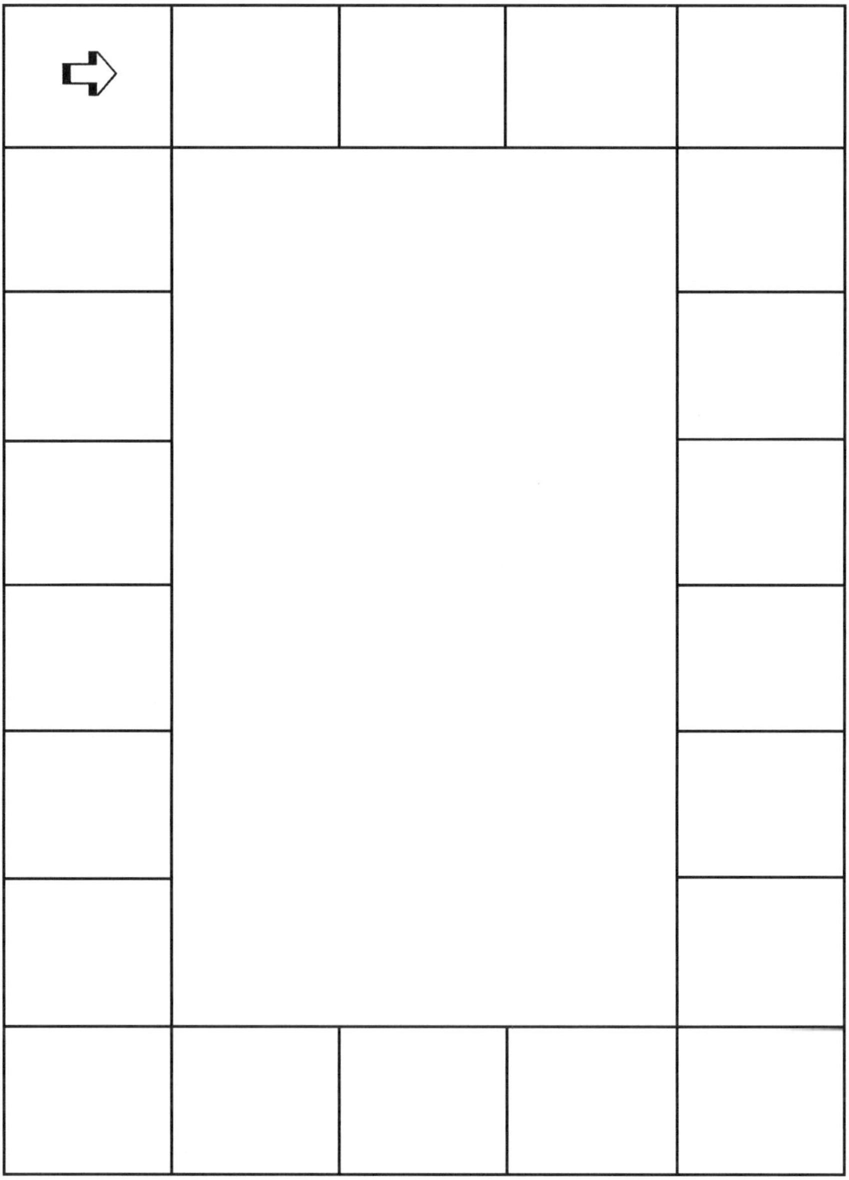

Fig. A24.2 Form for designing a board game

Design Our Board Game

Theme _____

Title of the game _____

Purpose

1. _____

2. _____

3. _____

Rules and procedures

1. _____

2. _____

3. _____

Symbols used
Questions asked

Fig. A24.3 Game board for individual session

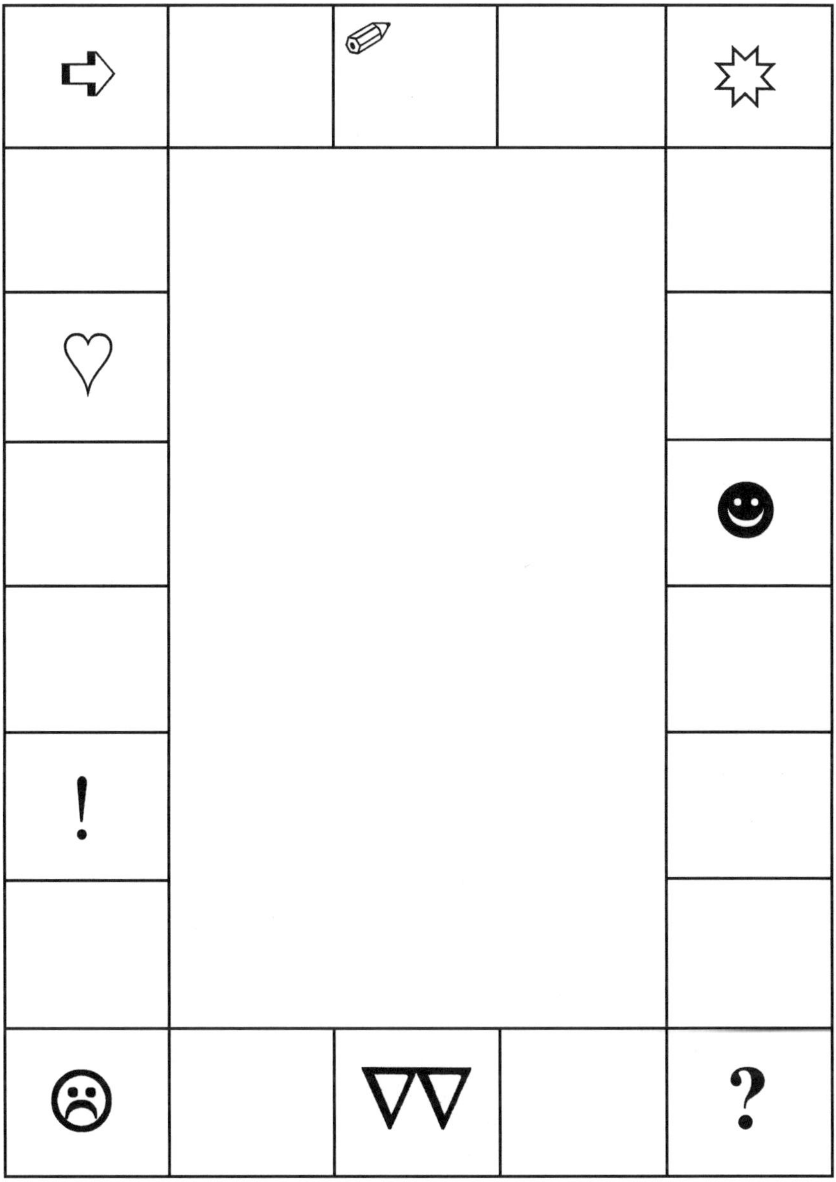

A25
Facing Divorce Feelings
Ed Muldrow

Items Needed

Feeling-faces cards (enlarge five copies of figure 3, and cut into squares)

Target Population

Children 7 and up or adults

Children, adolescents, or adults who have experienced divorce and have difficulties in talking about their feelings regarding the divorce

All cultures and socioeconomic backgrounds

Purpose

To help clients express and explore feelings of divorce and separation

To assess important grief stages and events in a client's life for future individual or group sessions

Procedure

Have clients sit in a circle. Explain the purpose of the game, and encourage clients to share their feelings about the divorce—past and current—and how they would like to feel about it in the future. Explain that there is no winner or loser in this game.

Shuffle the cards and deal five cards face down to each player. Place the remaining cards face down in the center.

The players should look for matches among their cards. A face with no eyes and mouth can be matched with any other feeling. Tell the players that when they have a matched pair of feeling cards, they will read the feeling out loud and describe that feeling as it applies to their situation. For example, "I feel sad when I leave my mom's house to visit my dad."

If a player does not have any matches, she or he should pick a card in the center and wait for the next turn. Alternatively, the player may pick any two feeling cards and discuss the mixed feelings she or he has.

Function in Assessment and Treatment

Assessment

This game is recommended for the beginning stages of therapy. It serves as a group or individual tool to help clients identify and express feelings. It also helps assess clients' problems and/or mixed feelings about their involvement in the divorce process.

Treatment

You can work with clients individually or in a group to better understand both the unique and common issues among family members coping with divorce. You can also use the identified feelings to process emotional responses and psychological resistance in order to help clients mediate conflict relationships with their family members. Ask follow-up questions to help clients process their feelings in an individual session. For example, "You mentioned that you felt really angry with your dad. What are some constructive ways you can express your anger?"

A26
Feelings Bingo
Jolene L. Pothier

Items Needed

Numbered bingo cards with incomplete sentences in each square (see figs. A26.1–4); use blank sheets [figs. A26.5–8] to make additional cards for small groups); tokens; set of numbers from 1 to 25 (make from a copy of fig. A26.9)

Target Population

Children or adults

Groups or families

Purpose

To break the ice

To build rapport

To help clients express and share their feelings

Procedure

Give each player a numbered bingo card and tokens. Tell players to cover the free space with a token. Select a number from the set of numbers and say it aloud. If players have the number on their cards, they should cover that space with a token.

Follow one of these procedures.

1. Clients who have the number on their bingo card must complete the sentence in that space.

2. Periodically have clients complete the sentence in that space. For example, on one turn have everyone place a token on the space, but not complete the sentence. With the next number, have everyone complete the sentence in his or her square.

3. Have clients take turns speaking each time a number is picked, one person per number.

Continue playing until someone has covered a row of five numbers on the bingo card in any direction—vertically, horizontally, or diagonally.

Function in Assessment and Treatment

Assessment

Use this game as a beginning game in a group session, particularly with families, to allow clients to express feelings in a nonthreatening atmosphere. Clients can disclose as much or as little as they want. Their responses may uncover needs, wants, likes, dislikes, strengths, weaknesses, and specific problems, which may be explored further, perhaps in individual sessions. The sentences in this game can be constructed to assess a specific type of situation or problem.

Treatment

This game helps clients understand and express themselves through feelings. During the game, you could ask a client to elaborate on his or her statement. This game is an excellent way to stimulate group discussion in a family, whether between parents and children, between siblings, or among the family as a whole. You could use follow-up questions to identify possible solutions to some common problems. For example, "You mentioned you hate to lose your temper. When was the last time that happened? How did you or others around you cope with the situation? How did you feel afterward?"

Fig. A26.1 Bingo card with numbers, version 1

1–5	6–10	11–15	16–20	21–25
B	**I**	**N**	**G**	**O**
I get angry when... 3	People can hurt my feelings by... 7	If I had a magic wand, I would... 15	I need more... 17	The best time of day for me is... 25
I would be happier if... 1	I wish I could... 6	I get sad when... 11	One of the best things about me is... 16	I once got hurt when... 24
I wish people would stop... 2	Once someone helped me by... 10	**FREE**	I don't like it when... 18	My family likes to... 23
A sound I like to hear is... 4	An important person to me is... 9	I would hate to lose... 14	I love to give... 19	If I could be invisible, I would... 22
I feel embarrassed when... 5	I get attention by... 8	An important thing in my life is... 12	Something I do well is... 20	I would like a great big... 21

Fig. A26.2 Bingo card with numbers, version 2

1–5	6–10	11–15	16–20	21–25
B	I	N	G	O
I get angry when... 2	People can hurt my feelings by... 8	If I had a magic wand, I would... 11	I need more... 16	The best time of day for me is... 21
I would be happier if... 5	I wish I could... 10	I get sad when... 15	One of the best things about me is... 20	I once got hurt when... 25
I wish people would stop... 4	Once someone helped me by... 9	FREE	I don't like it when... 17	My family likes to... 22
A sound I like to hear is... 3	An important person to me is... 6	I would hate to lose... 13	I love to give... 18	If I could be invisible, I would... 24
I feel embarrassed when... 1	I get attention by... 7	An important thing in my life is... 14	Something I do well is... 19	I would like a great big... 23

Fig. A26.3 Bingo card with numbers, version 3

1–5	6–10	11–15	16–20	21–25
B	**I**	**N**	**G**	**O**
I get angry when...	People can hurt my feelings by...	If I had a magic wand, I would...	I need more...	The best time of day for me is...
4	6	13	19	22
I would be happier if...	I wish I could...	I get sad when...	One of the best things about me is...	I once got hurt when...
3	8	12	18	23
I wish people would stop...	Once someone helped me by...	**FREE**	I don't like it when...	My family likes to...
1	7		16	21
A sound I like to hear is...	An important person to me is...	I would hate to lose...	I love to give...	If I could be invisible, I would...
5	10	15	20	25
I feel embarrassed when...	I get attention by...	An important thing in my life is...	Something I do well is...	I would like a great big...
2	9	14	17	24

Fig. A26.4 Bingo card with numbers, version 4

1–5	6–10	11–15	16–20	21–25
B	**I**	**N**	**G**	**O**
I get angry when... 5	People can hurt my feelings by... 10	If I had a magic wand, I would... 12	I need more... 20	The best time of day for me is... 23
I would be happier if... 2	I wish I could... 9	I get sad when... 13	One of the best things about me is... 17	I once got hurt when... 22
I wish people would stop... 4	Once someone helped me by... 8	**FREE**	I don't like it when... 19	My family likes to... 24
A sound I like to hear is... 1	An important person to me is... 7	I would hate to lose... 11	I love to give... 16	If I could be invisible, I would... 21
I feel embarrassed when... 3	I get attention by... 6	An important thing in my life is... 15	Something I do well is... 18	I would like a great big... 25

Fig. A26.5 Bingo card without numbers, version 1

1–5	6–10	11–15	16–20	21–25
B	**I**	**N**	**G**	**O**
I get angry when...	People can hurt my feelings by...	If I had a magic wand, I would...	I need more...	The best time of day for me is...
I would be happier if...	I wish I could...	I get sad when...	One of the best things about me is...	I once got hurt when...
I wish people would stop...	Once someone helped me by...	**FREE**	I don't like it when...	My family likes to...
A sound I like to hear is...	An important person to me is...	I would hate to lose...	I love to give...	If I could be invisible, I would...
I feel embarrassed when...	I get attention by...	An important thing in my life is...	Something I do well is...	I would like a great big...

Fig. A26.6 Bingo card without numbers, version 2

1–5	6–10	11–15	16–20	21–25
B	I	N	G	O
People can hurt my feelings by...	I get angry when...	If I had a magic wand, I would...	I need more...	The best time of day for me is...
I wish I could...	I would be happier if...	I get sad when...	One of the best things about me is...	I once got hurt when...
Once someone helped me by...	I wish people would stop...	FREE	I don't like it when...	My family likes to...
An important person to me is...	A sound I like to hear is...	I would hate to lose...	I love to give...	If I could be invisible, I would...
I get attention by...	I feel embarrassed when...	An important thing in my life is...	Something I do well is...	I would like a great big...

Fig. A26.7 Bingo card without numbers, version 3

1–5	6–10	11–15	16–20	21–25
B	I	N	G	O
I get angry when...	I need more...	If I had a magic wand, I would...	People can hurt my feelings by...	The best time of day for me is...
I would be happier if...	One of the best things about me is...	I get sad when...	I wish I could...	I once got hurt when...
I wish people would stop...	I don't like it when...	FREE	Once someone helped me by...	My family likes to...
A sound I like to hear is...	I love to give...	I would hate to lose...	An important person to me is...	If I could be invisible, I would...
I feel embarrassed when...	Something I do well is...	An important thing in my life is...	I get attention by...	I would like a great big...

Fig. A26.8 Bingo card without numbers, version 4

1–5	6–10	11–15	16–20	21–25
B	I	N	G	O
I get angry when...	People can hurt my feelings by...	If I had a magic wand, I would...	The best time of day for me is...	I need more...
I would be happier if...	I wish I could...	I get sad when...	I once got hurt when...	One of the best things about me is...
I wish people would stop...	Once someone helped me by...	FREE	My family likes to...	I don't like it when...
A sound I like to hear is...	An important person to me is...	I would hate to lose...	If I could be invisible, I would...	I love to give...
I feel embarrassed when...	I get attention by...	An important thing in my life is...	I would like a great big...	Something I do well is...

Fig. A26.9 Bingo numbers

1	2	3	4	5
6	7	8	9	10
11	12	13	14	15
16	17	18	19	20
21	22	23	24	25

A27
Follow-Me Story
Monit Cheung

Items Needed

A box of playing cards or any creative game cards. For very young children or children with developmental difficulties, use cards with pictures instead of playing cards (Creative Child Games makes several different sets of picture cards).

Target Population

Children 6 and up or adults

All cultures and socioeconomic backgrounds

Purpose

To break the ice

To build rapport

To assess free-association skills

Procedure

Shuffle the cards and deal five cards to each person facedown. Place the remaining cards in the deck facedown on the table. Turn the top card in the deck over and state the title of a story based on the symbol or number on the card. For ♥5 it could be "A Happy Princess with Five Happy Wishes," "Five Days before Christmas," or "A Story about Five Brothers and Sisters," for example.

Place one card on the table and begin the first line of the story. For ♦K it could be "Once upon a time, there was an old king living in a palace far away."

Prompt the player to your right to continue the story by putting down a card and using a clue from the last line. For example, ♣A, "His palace has a tree with black fruit." If players cannot think of a line to follow, allow them to say "pass."

Before discarding the last card, players have to say, "Follow me." Otherwise, they either draw one card from the pile or pretend to be one of the characters in the story by making some noise.

The player who holds the last card of the game ends the story.

Function in Assessment and Treatment

Assessment

This game is a rapport-building tool. It serves as a beginning game in a group session. You could use it in individual sessions before discussing serious matters, to help clients relax and guide them in a nonthreatening way to talk about their problems. Also, it allows clients to exercise their imagination while helping you assess their capacity for free association. In general, using the story-telling technique can create a safe place for clients to share their views (Brandell, 1988).

Treatment

Use words such as "difficulty," "secret," "question," "idea," "opinion," "know what to do," etc., to guide clients (especially nonverbal ones) to talk more about their perceived solution. Here is an example.

♠2 The prince found it difficult to talk and asked the two rabbits to help him.

♦J The rabbits had a secret passageway that they could use to help the prince.

♥8 The prince didn't know this secret but wanted to know it from the bottom of his heart.

♣4 But the rabbits ran away with four gold coins.

♦10 One coin fell, and it told the prince how to get inside the passageway.

Hot Potato Game

Sharon Clark Peska

Items Needed

Hot Potato by Hasbro; 2 AAA batteries; 12 game cards (one set designed for children and one set designed for adolescents/adults; see table A28.1)

Target Population

Children 3 and up or adults

Clients who have difficulties talking about their emotions and/or past experience

Two or more players

Purpose

To break the ice

To build rapport

To encourage expressing feelings

Procedure

Caution: Use this exercise in the beginning process of disclosure. It should not be used to get into deep discussion about a person's past.

Choose between the child Hot Potato cards and the adolescent/adult cards. Sit on the floor or at a table, or stand in a circle. Place the Hot Potato cards picture-side up in the middle of your playing area.

Prompt the first player to start the game by holding the potato head and squeezing it (music should start). Instruct players to pass or toss the potato from player to player. Be sure that they keep the Hot Potato moving.

When the music stops and the potato says, "Yahoo," the player caught with the Hot Potato collects one card. If the Hot Potato was in midair when he said, "Yahoo," the player who just released him collects the card.

The player reads the emotion out loud and describes that feeling as it applies to him or her. For example, if the player picks the emotion sad, the player says "sad" and then proceeds with "I feel sad when my mom drinks too much," or "I am sad today because I miss my brother." The player can choose to elaborate, or you may ask a few questions to gain more information. The player can also choose not to go into any more detail.

After players finish disclosing their emotion, they hand the Hot Potato to the person on the left. The new player squeezes the potato and resumes the game.

The player who collects the most Hot Potato cards receives a prize.

Function in Assessment and Treatment

Assessment

This game is a group tool that allows clients to begin the process of disclosure. It also allows clients to trust each other, if they are prompted to respect each other's statements and to maintain confidentiality. This game can increase your insight into clients' problems.

Treatment

Probe clients about what was mentioned in the activity in order to gain greater understanding and insight. For example, ask, "During the game you mentioned feeling upset because of your brother. Tell me more. What do you do to cope with this feeling?" You can also process with the client how he or she felt during the game, and decide the next step in therapy.

Table A28.1   Game cards for Hot Potato

For children	For adolescents and adults
Excited	Excited
Stirred-up	Aroused, stirred-up
Stimulated	Stimulated
Silly	Pleased
Foolish	Delighted
Not serious	Content
Loving	Loving
Able to care	Able to care
Warmhearted	Warmhearted
Interested	Interested
Curious	Curious
Paying attention	Paying attention
Surprised	Smart
Blown away	Intelligent
Shocked	Stylish
Happy	Happy
Great pleasure	Great pleasure
Joyful	Joyful
Angry	Angry
Mad	Mad
Upset	Upset
Shy	Stressed
Bashful	Anxious
Distrustful	Feeling pressured
Lonely	Depressed
Alone	Sad or gloomy
Empty	Low spirits
Frightened	Disappointed
Scared	Dissatisfied with hopes
Jumpy	or expectations
Cranky	Guilty
Crouchy	Blameworthy
Grumpy	Found at fault
Confused	Confused
Mixed-up	Mixed-up
Not able to understand	Not able to understand

Incomplete Sentences

Monit Cheung

Items Needed

35 small index cards (3" × 5"); 10 large index cards (4" × 6")

Target Population

Children or adults with specific issues or problems such as eating disorder

All cultures and socioeconomic backgrounds

Purpose

To help clients free-associate any feelings related to prior experiences, such as eating disorder, divorce, or separation

To identify the source of these feelings

To encourage clients to talk about their emotional responses toward these feelings

To assess client strengths

Procedure

Copy the game cards (table A29.1), cut each sentence out and paste it on a small index card. Print words from the question/comment cards (table A29.2) on the bigger index cards. For group therapy, use two sets of the game cards.

In an individual session, take turns with the client answering each of the incomplete sentences. Based on the information provided after five rounds, place the first question/comment card on the table and ask a question or make a comment regarding the client's strengths. The client will also ask a question or make a comment regarding your strengths. In subsequent rounds, the question/comment cards can be related to identifying problems, locating resources, finding solutions, or other thoughts.

In a group or family session, ask clients to pay attention to the completed sentences. After all sentences have been completed, encourage each individual to ask a question or make a comment based on what he or she has heard. For example,

1. When you said [completing the sentence], what did it mean?
2. When you said _____, how did you feel? How do you feel now?
3. You said you were scared when you _____; what else would scare you?
4. You said that your father _____; tell me more about it.

This question or comment can be addressed to the individual who has just completed a sentence, or to another individual who is related to the information given. If the individual who was asked the question does not want to answer, this individual will pick another sentence to complete.

Function in Assessment and Treatment

Assessment

This free-association activity allows clients to address any issue or problem (Meyer, 1991). At the same time, it assesses clients' potential and strengths in resolving problems or reaching conclusions.

Treatment

This activity applies a balanced perspective to help clients realize that everybody has problems as well as strengths to solve them. Additional incomplete sentences can be added to draw clients' attention to making decisions, finding alternatives, and consulting with friends and family. It is noted that although the first two rounds may generate only surface information about clients, your encouragement and direct involvement can make this activity a therapeutic tool. It is important that clients be encouraged to ask simple questions and are attentive to their own problem-solving potential. Add specific activity cards to reflect the client's specific problems, strengths, or solutions. In the case of eating disorder, examples can include: "I look at this problem seriously because . . ." "I eat a lot when I feel . . ." "When I feel like eating after a full meal, I will . . ." "When I have a problem, I would like to discuss the solution with . . ." "I am a person good at . . ."

Table A29.1 Game cards for Incomplete Sentences

When I am sad . . .	I feel scared when . . .
People like to . . .	I consider myself . . .
It's so easy to . . .	If I were a man (woman), I would . . .
I'd like to let go . . .	My mother is . . .
My greatest talent is . . .	I'm the type of person who . . .
I'm concerned about . . .	When I feel happy, I . . .
I can get really mad when . . .	It's so hard to . . .
I need to . . .	My friends always . . .
Most of all I want . . .	I cannot stand it when . . .
I was punished when . . .	I have fun when . . .
My father is . . .	My partner always . . .
I think of myself as . . .	I am afraid . . .
I feel comfortable when . . .	The best day of my life was . . .
My greatest weakness is . . .	When a person is angry, he or she will . . .
I had a bad dream about . . .	I really care about . . .
I like to . . .	I am so confused because . . .
Women are . . .	I am confident that . . .
One of my wishes is . . .	

Table A29.2 Question/comment cards

Strengths

Problems

Resources

Solutions

Other thoughts

A30
Journal of Feelings
Monit Cheung

Items Needed

A 40-page notebook; 2 sheets of colored paper (8½" × 11")

Target Population

Children and their families with communication issues

All cultures and socioeconomic backgrounds

Purpose

To build rapport

To help both children and parents identify and understand the role and impact of good and bad feelings

To provide a means to enhance communication between parents and children and to promote mutual understanding

Procedure

Use the notebook as a journal for the family. Help the family design a cover page for the good-feelings journal, with a happy face and the title "Things That Make Me Feel Good." Have them design another cover page for the bad-feelings journal, with a sad face and the title "Things That Make Me Feel Bad." Paste the happy page on the front cover of the notebook and the sad page upside down on the back cover.

On each page inside the notebook, draw a line to separate it into two halves. Label them "Children" and "Parents." Every day, for at least two weeks, instruct both children and parents to fill a page for the good-feelings journal, and then to flip it over and fill a page for the bad-feelings journal. Clients may write, draw, or paste in photographs or pictures from newspapers or magazines. Tell them to date each entry.

Instruct clients to share the feelings every day with a family member at a preset time, for example, for ten minutes after dinner. Tell them to bring the journal to every session to share with you.

Function in Assessment and Treatment

Assessment

This activity is adapted from an activity designed by L. E. Shapiro (1993) as a game to help children build self-esteem. It is modified to enhance communication between parents and their children. The journal contents can be used as an assessment tool in a therapeutic session. It is important to note that some parents may pressure children to express what the parents want to hear. Similarly, children may write what they think their parents want to see. Assess the parents' commitment to enhancing communication, and explain to children about the parents' intent to learn their feelings. If necessary, separate the journals into a children's journal and a parents' journal, which will be revealed to each other only after you assess whether that is suitable.

Treatment

Encourage the family members to tell one another about what they drew, wrote, or expressed in the good-feelings and bad-feelings journals. The family can also create a collage (a magazine cut-and-paste activity) during the session to relate to their discussions. This activity can be modified for use in a non-family group setting. It is important that feelings are analyzed with specific examples or family situations. The session can also include individual written responses to the journals, for additional comments regarding this exercise.

Me on the Outside and the Inside

Molly Grimmer

Items Needed

Shoe boxes with lids; construction paper; scissors; glue, tape, stapler, markers, crayons, paint, glitter; craft supplies such as ribbons, cotton balls, sequins, stickers, twine, fabric, magazines, small trinkets, beads.

Target Population

Groups of children and adolescents (6 and older), or families with issues that have not been disclosed

All cultures and socioeconomic backgrounds

Purpose

To build rapport

To help facilitate discussion of feelings

To help clients identify their feelings and learn that it is normal to have a variety of feelings

To help clients understand that the way you look and act on the outside does not always match how you feel on the inside

Procedure

This activity takes two sessions. You keep the box between sessions.

Give each participant a shoe box and access to art and craft supplies. Prompt participants to decorate the outside of the box as they feel others see them from the outside, and to decorate the inside of the box as they feel on the inside.

Once the boxes are complete, have participants describe the outside of their box and discuss how they feel others perceive them. Tell them to describe how they decorated the inside of their box. Encourage participants to share the symbolism of the decorations. Ask questions and encourage participants to talk about the feelings associated with each of the decorations.

This activity was used in Family Service Center's (FSC) Incest Treatment Program in Houston in the mid- to late 1980s with groups of sexually abused girls.

After talking about the completed boxes, prompt participants to discuss how they felt while making the box, and how they felt after sharing their feelings. Assess if these feelings are similar or different from the feelings decorated on the box.

Function in Assessment and Treatment

Assessment

This activity is primarily a treatment tool; however, clients' self-image and perception of unresolved feelings can also be assessed.

Treatment

The activity provides insight for participants into their "hidden" feelings. It provides an opportunity for identification and discussion about feelings. This is a great activity to allow for creative expression and the client's own interpretation. In a group session, ask each client to describe the meaning of each of the symbols used in the box and share how these meanings may be related to how other people see them. In an individual session, ask additional questions to help the client to process his or her feelings, such as, "Let's talk about what's on the inside of your box? How do you feel when you have feelings or experiences that cannot be shared?"

Memory Chain

Sandra A. Lopez

Items Needed

Construction paper of different colors (8½" × 11"); transparent tape, glue, or stapler; markers; scissors

Target Population

Children 7 to 12

Individual child, family, or group of children

Purpose

To help clients express grief about the loss of a loved one

To help clients have a safe outlet for remembering or noting memories about a loved one who has died

To teach clients about the need for remembering loved ones after they have died

To provide a symbolic remembrance that can be shared with other family members

Procedure

Encourage the client to pick several colors of construction paper. Help the client cut the paper into ten (or more) strips 8½" long and 1½" wide.

Encourage the client to think of memories he or she may have about the loved one who passed away, and to write these memories on the individual pieces of construction paper. For example, "Sue liked pizza," "Sue played games with me," "Sue was mean sometimes but I listened to her."

Help the client glue, tape, or staple the strips together to make a chain. Once all pieces are linked together, encourage the client to share these memories and talk about how these memories affect him or her. Suggest that the client hang the memory chain in a special place at home.

Function in Assessment and Treatment

Assessment

Use this activity to encourage clients to remember and talk about special memories they have of loved ones who have died. Clients are free to disclose positive as well as negative memories of their loved one, so as to portray a realistic picture. Their memories may provide significant material for you to explore in future sessions. For example, the client's responses may indicate areas for exploration of potential unresolved grief issues, or complicated grief that involves other family members or other individual and family factors.

Treatment

This activity helps clients understand that it is important to remember their loved ones, to talk about them, to discuss the good and bad memories they may have, and to receive validation of these memories from the therapist. In group situations, children can relate to other children's grief stories. In family therapy, adults may begin to understand the child's grief as well.

Mixed Feelings
Monit Cheung

Items Needed

Colored markers; tokens or other small items in a container; feeling-faces (fig. 3); 20 pieces of paper (2" × 3")

Target Population

Children or adults with mixed feelings toward a particular incident or event

Purpose

To help clients express ambivalent and contradictory feelings

To help clients understand it is normal to experience different kinds of feelings toward the same incident

Procedure

Begin by asking clients to write down and draw different kinds of feelings they often have (from the feeling-faces pictures or other sources) on the small pieces of paper.

Give an example to initiate a sense of joining. Make feeling cards by drawing feeling faces or words, each on a small piece of paper (e.g., aggressive, angry, anxious, confident, embarrassed, happy, hurt, lonely, loved, pained, proud, shocked, shy, surprised); these cards can be made in advance or during the session. Tell a personal story and put the tokens or small items on the feeling cards whenever that feeling is mentioned. The more small items placed on the feeling, the stronger that feeling was. The same feeling can be repeated in the story. For example, "Two months ago, I had a car accident. I was completely *shocked* [put five items on this feeling card], and felt *pain* [three items] in my chest. After I managed to get my car to a complete stop, I realized I couldn't open the door. I just sat there, wondering what I should do next. I guess I was *shocked* [two more items], and I couldn't think straight. A man came to my window and checked if I was all right. Suddenly, I felt *anxious* [four items] and *lonely* [three items], and just wanted to call my husband. The moment that my husband arrived, I cried—I must have felt *released* [add this feeling card and put ten items on it]. I was extremely *happy* [seven items] that he came immediately to help me."

After giving an example, direct each client to tell a personal story with feeling words, and to put items on the feeling cards to show the intensity of each feeling. For younger children, the story can be constructed first and feeling words added later.

After the story, help the client comment on his or her current feelings (not past feelings) toward that incident.

Function in Assessment and Treatment

Assessment

This exercise assesses clients' ability to conceptualize and relate feelings to a concrete situation. It also helps you identify specific feelings that clients can't express well.

Treatment

This game enables clients to name a variety of feelings. It is an educational tool to help clients understand that all feelings are valuable and relevant, and that many feelings can be involved in any given situation. This game also helps clients feel confident in their ability to understand and express themselves, and can help individuals process complex emotional reactions. For example, this game can be used to help teenagers process parent-child relationship issues that elicit mixed emotional responses.

Name Associations

Monit Cheung

Items Needed

2 sheets of paper (8½" × 11") for each person; transparent tape

Target Population

Children, adolescents, or adults for self-image building

Any language

Purpose

To break the ice

To help clients introduce themselves in a nonthreatening way

To identify issues or problems associated with this activity

Procedure

Distribute two sheets of paper to each client.

Ask clients to write their first name vertically in all capital letters along the left edge of the first sheet of paper. Encourage them to make large letters, spaced so that the entire sheet of paper is used (fig. A34.1).

Ask clients to think of words that begin with (or contain) each of the letters in their name. These words should describe some aspects of their personality, likes or dislikes, and so forth. Use your name as an example (figs. A34.2, A34.3).

Within a minute or two, have each person introduce himself or herself with some or all the words written on their sheet, for example, "My name is Monit. I am a motivated individual. I like the color orange, but I am allergic to oranges. I am neat, and I always take the initiative to talk with others. I like to be with my family and get a sense of togetherness."

In a group meeting, after each person introduces himself or herself, this sheet can be taped next to the individual (in front of a desk or on the wall) as a name-plate for the session

Function in Assessment and Treatment

Assessment

Name games are common icebreakers in group meetings. Morris and Fritz (2002) suggest modifying name games so that each participant will focus on the social nature of recall. In this activity, the use of the client's name to associate with some social aspects of this individual will help break the ice. You can assess clients' willingness to describe themselves. If individuals refuse to participate or do not have any words to associate with their characteristics, ask them to write down any words as a start. If you sense negativity, talk with these clients individually about self-description and self-image. Clients' lack of participation could be a lack of motivation to join the group.

Treatment

Use this exercise as a treatment tool for clients to free-associate words about their problems and the solutions they may have undertaken. Each time this exercise is used, record a date on the sheet, and put it in the client's file for future comparisons. Usually the words chosen at an initial meeting are more generic and positive. As treatment progresses, more word choices may be discovered. If using a solution-focused approach for treatment, you may choose to use this exercise to encourage clients to identify various ways of dealing with the identified problem.

Suggested themes for designing the name sheet in ten sessions can be

1. Your characteristics or something representing yourself
2. Your perceptions about your family
3. Your way of dealing with anxiety
4. An introduction to your significant others or friends
5. Your problems or your family problems
6. Your potential and strengths
7. Strengths of your family
8. Solutions for your problem
9. A few wishes that you would like to come true
10. Feelings associated with therapy

Fig. A34.1 Starting card for Name Associations

M
O
N
I
T

Fig. A34.2 Sample of completed card, with words starting with each letter

Motivated
Orange
Neat
Initiative
Together

Fig. A34.3 Sample of completed card, with words containing each letter

Motivated
tOgetherness
Neat
bIg dream
Teacher

A35

Paper Bombs

Monit Cheung

Items Needed

A sheet of 8½" × 11" paper for each participant; permanent markers (various colors); 1 or 2 water buckets half-filled with water; paper towels; masking tape

Target Population

Children 3–12

Hyperactive children or developmentally delayed children

Groups of 5–10 children, adolescents, and family members

Purpose

To help clients release anger and/or frustration in a safe way

Procedure

This game may be perceived as too violent in certain cultures or belief systems. Use it with caution, provide adequate guidance, and model appropriate behavior.

Ask clients to draw a large picture of the target person (e.g., an abuser, a person representing a specific disease, an irresponsible person, etc.). Tell them to draw an outline first, then add facial expression.

Ask, "Are there any other body parts you would like to add?"

Tape the drawing on a wall about the height of the client. In a group setting, remind clients not to tape the drawings too close together.

Wet three pieces of paper towels and roll them loosely like a ball.

Ask the client to stand two feet in front of the drawing. Instruct the client to throw a paper ball at the drawing.

Give the client a second ball. Ask him or her to say, "You are not treating me right!" or something the client feels about this symbolic target.

Encourage the client to say it louder before throwing the third ball.

Discuss feelings with the client.

Function in Assessment and Treatment

Assessment

Children tend to internalize feelings when they do not know how to express them (Fischetti, 2001). This game helps you assess clients' level of frustration so you can educate clients on the importance of expressing feelings to release their anxiety.

Treatment

Clients can learn how to deal with their anger or frustrations in a controlled environment. After this game, help hyperactive children identify ways to deal with their excessive energy at home. Children can also invite their parents to the next session to witness their "bombing," so that their parents can talk about children's needs to express frustration. This game helps children who have been abused express their anger and share their mixed feelings toward the abuser or the nonsupportive parent. Since this game may involve excessive energy, debriefing should include questions such as "When you threw your bombs, what did you think of?" "Since you cannot throw things at others, this game is used only in this room to help you process your feeling. What would be an appropriate way in school (or at home) to express your frustration and anger?"

Red Bead Success

Barbara J. Brandes

Items Needed

12" length of thread for stringing beads for each person; red beads (equivalent to 9" per person); two to three times as many assorted beads as red beads (the more distracting or alluring the assorted beads, the better); zip bags or bowls

Target Population

Ages 13 and up

Groups

Purpose

To break the ice

To develop awareness of self (strengths and weaknesses when presented with choices)

To strengthen ability to assess risks and make decisions based on goals

To develop understanding of social conflicts and self-determination

To develop willingness to explore positives and negatives of peer influence and the role of self-determination in the selection of friends

Procedure

You can tie one red bead to the string to start each bracelet. Put beads into a separate container (such as zip bags) for each participant, or put them into one container (such as a bowl) for each group of three to five participants. Each container should have enough red beads so that each participant can make a red bead bracelet, and enough assorted beads to tempt each participant to make a unique bracelet. Make a sample bracelet all of red beads.

Tell the group that at some of the temples in China, they can purchase a red bead bracelet to remind them to remain focused on the meditations of their heart. Show them a red bead bracelet to emphasize the point.

Explain to the group, "I want each of you to create a red bead bracelet, so that it can remind you to stay focused on the goals you set for yourself today. Let's call it a success bracelet." Tell the group how long they can work on the bracelets, until they are completed or for a certain period of time, if you are under a time constraint.

Begin to distribute the beads, but say (as if surprised), "Oh, we have some different colors and types of beads. I wonder how your bracelet will come out," or "Oops! Sorry about that. This is kind of like life, where there are really lots of choices and ways to express yourself." If asked specifically whether the other beads can be used, try to avoid eliminating the opportunity for self-determination. Make a nonemphatic statement such as, "That's your decision," while making statements during the process such as, "You really seem to be attracted to the pink beads," or "Wow! That might be the bracelet with the most fish/silver beads/hearts/etc."

When the bracelets are completed, or when the time is up, tell participants, "Let's look at our success [pause]. How many red beads did each of you use to make your success bracelet?" To promote participation, it is helpful to use a chalk board or poster to write down the number of red beads that were used by each participant (names of participants do not need to be written on the board). Emphasize that "success" in this game is the number of red beads, but that this game is like life.

Discuss the distractions of the assorted beads, contrasting and comparing the selection of beads to the selection of activities or pursuits in life. Active involvement of participants is important. Encourage participation in the discussion by asking specific questions such as, "What kind of activities might the sparkly beads represent?" "What are you most tempted to go and do instead of studying? What color bead might that be in your bracelet?"

Ask participants to share with the group something about what they learned today from playing this game. Encourage participants to keep the bead bracelet as a symbol of what was learned.

Function in Assessment and Treatment

Assessment

This game helps clients identify situations that lead to unnecessarily risky behavior or to poor decision making. It allows participants to explore group temptations and concepts of peer pressure, and gives you an insight into varying degrees of vulnerability to peer pressure as evidenced by participants in the game. If the game becomes too competitive and leads to excessive arguments, stop it and help participants process their feelings.

Treatment

Use comparisons related to specific, relevant treatment issues, such as the temptation to go drinking with friends rather than attending an alcohol-free event at a classmate's house. You can also solicit comparisons from participants to encourage them to identify the triggers for the behavior they want to change. The discussion can create a safe place for self-disclosure and to guide participants toward greater understanding of their perceived situations, including choices, potential consequences, and value-laden alternatives or objectives.

A37
Sand Play
Monit Cheung

Items Needed

Tray, wood or plastic (22.5" × 28.5" × 3"), with the inside bottom painted blue; fine sand or rice; toys or materials on shelf or next to tray.

Animals: domestic cat, dog, goldfish; wild elephant, tiger, lion, rabbit, deer, dinosaur, shark, whale, octopus; farm animals: chicken, cow, sheep, horse, pig

Balls: tennis, miniature football, miniature basketball

Barriers: fences, screens, signs

Blocks or plastic bricks

Buildings: bridge, castle, house, igloo

Family figures: male, female, girl, boy, baby, people of color

Fantasy figures: fairytale and cartoon figures, king and queen, prince and princess, magician, witch or wizard, dragon, unicorn, Kirin

Fighting figures (plastic): soldiers, gun, knife, knights, sword

Furniture: bed, chairs and tables, refrigerator, sofa, TV set

Grooming items: comb and brush, unbreakable mirror

Historical figures: cowboys, saints, soldiers

Kitchen set: cooking utensil, plastic container, pot, pan, spoon, stove/oven

Monsters

Mountains, rock and cave, volcano

Musical instruments: drums, guitar, horn, piano

Plants: cactus, flowers, trees (deciduous and evergreen, full and bare), seaweed

Seashells, rocks, fossils

Skeleton, skull, bones (all plastic)

Spiritual: candles, figures from different religions (e.g., cross, gods, shrine)

Transportation: airplane, boat, car, fuel truck, police car, emergency/rescue vehicle, train

Miscellaneous: Band-Aid, crystal ball, tablecloth, colored paper, feather, jewel, unbreakable lightbulb, mask, snowflake, star

Target Population

Clients of all ages who have been resistant to therapy

Victims of sexual abuse

Groups or families

Purpose

To help clients express themselves in a safe environment

To assess the developmental stage, capabilities, motor skills, strengths, problems of the client

To help the group define the identifying problem(s)

To assist the therapy in the development of a treatment plan

To therapeutically relate to clients' world

Procedure

Place the toys and other materials around the tray.

Ask the client to choose five to ten items and place them in the tray. In group settings, ask each person to choose five and take turns to place one item at a time in the tray. Spell out the rules: Don't throw sand on floor, don't break objects, and don't put sand or toys in mouth, nose, eyes, or ears.

Do not interpret the sand tray, but encourage clients to tell a story about the image projected by the items in the tray.

Take a photo of the completed project for comparison and treatment purposes. Don't remove any items from the sand tray in front of clients without asking. Encourage clients to remove the items and put them back on the shelf, if necessary.

Function in Assessment and Treatment

Assessment

Sand-tray therapy is an effective way to allow clients to express their feelings, thoughts, and emotions in a safe way (Mitchell & Friedman, 1994). In group therapy, each item can relate to other group members in some meaningful ways (Allan & Berry, 2002). Encourage clients, after placing the item on the tray, to think about the relationship of this item to the target problem, stated emotions, or the group, in order to assess clients' definition of the problem and their relationship with others.

Treatment

Although sand play is considered a free-association game, it can be used as a structural storytelling game if you start with an introduction or a theme. After setting a goal, each client may choose items to complete a story in order to achieve that goal. Solutions may come from the items when you ask therapeutically related questions, such as the following:

1. How does this item remind you of a strategy that you are you planning to use to encounter the problem?
2. What alternative method may we adopt to help this family detour from the current situation?
3. Where would this family go if this item weren't a part of this story?
4. What did you do that could solve the problem?
5. How does this item relate to any other items in the tray (or outside of the tray)?
6. Who would you talk to if you faced some barriers in this journey?
7. How does this sand tray relate to the actual situation that you and your family are dealing with now?

A38

Throwing Balls

Winnie W. Y. Chan

Items Needed

Tennis balls (10 balls per 5–10 people in a group)

Target Population

Children, adolescents, or adults (5 years and older)

Groups (10 per group)

Purpose

To break the ice

To address the issues of group communication

To help clients share their feelings regarding group communication

Procedure

Ask clients to stand in a circle. Begin by saying a client's name and tossing a tennis ball to that person. Instruct that person to announce the name of another client in the circle, and then to throw the ball to that person. Continue until everyone in the group has had a chance to throw and receive the ball.

In the second round, attempt to keep the same order of names, and repeat the exercise.

After repeating for several rounds, add another ball to the circle. Tell clients to toss this ball around the group in the same order as the first round. Add additional balls to the circle until the group cannot manage anymore.

After the game is over, ask clients to describe how they felt about the game or one thing they can learn from the game. If sufficient balls are available, give each client a ball during this debriefing period. After they provide some verbal feedback, instruct clients to throw the ball into a collection box. The following questions can be used to facilitate discussion:

1. What techniques are helpful when playing the game?

2. How do you feel as the person who throws the ball?

3. How do you feel as the person who receives the ball?

4. How do you feel as part of the group in this game?

5. How would you feel if you were outside this group?

6. What insights does this game give to you?

Function in Assessment and Treatment

Assessment

This game is not an assessment tool. It serves as a beginning game in a group session to help clients have fun before serious matters are discussed. Use the game to encourage clients to set up rules for the group in a nonthreatening way.

Treatment

If the game involves a group whose members have known each other for a while, use the debriefing questions to help clients share their feelings toward the group. You can also use the game to highlight the skills of group participation and communication, such as having eye contact and being sensitive to the recipient's response.

Wallpaper Feelings

Monit Cheung

Items Needed

Pieces of wallpaper of various patterns, colors, and sizes; wallpaper books if available; table or carpeted floor; scratch paper; pencils. Materials other than wallpaper, such as fabric, can be used. Choose different solids, patterns, colors, and designs (animals, flowers, toys) for different treatment purposes.

Target Population

Children, adolescents, or adults exploring feelings about their families

Groups of 10

Purpose

To break the ice

To help clients share their feelings

To help children design a room and address issues of privacy

Procedure

Icebreaker

Lay the wallpaper on a table or a carpeted floor. Ask clients to choose one piece of wallpaper. (Tell them it is OK to share.)

Ask them to look at the selected wallpaper for one minute and think of two words they associate with the paper. Take turns sharing what these two words are (or have clients write these words down and share).

Design a Room

Ask the client to pick the wallpaper he or she likes.

Ask the client to imagine he or she is using this wallpaper to design a room. Or ask him or her to draw a room and cut the wallpaper to decorate this room.

Encourage the client to talk about this room or share feelings about this room. Try the following questions:

1. Whose room is it?
2. What purpose does this room have?

3. What would you like to put in this room?

4. Whom would you invite to come for a first visit?

5. Whom would you rather *not* invite?

6. When would you use this room?

7. How long would you like to stay there?

8. Who would help you design your room?

9. How would you feel when you are inside/outside this room?

Function in Assessment and Treatment

Assessment

This icebreaker can also be used for free association. It can help you understand the child's definition of "my world."

Treatment

Use this exercise as a feeling-expression game. After the client picks a wallpaper, ask, "Look at the wallpaper and see what this paper has that can reflect how you feel today." It helps nonverbal clients express their feelings through free association.

Part B
Guided Imagery

Introduction

Natural healing philosophies focus on the mind-body connection, and their usage can be traced to ancient times. In modern Western society, however, there is often little acknowledgment of natural healing approaches. The complexity of human relationships, fast-paced lifestyle, polluted environments, tension-creating living, and our overstimulated minds constantly stress our physical and mental well-being. Returning to ancient tradition, many health and mental health professionals are urging individuals to naturally alter their lifestyles by spending more solitary time listening to their inner voice. The practice of meditation has been used for thousands of years in the Buddhist tradition to help people relax and focus, and modern applications of this contemplative practice are becoming increasingly accepted by the mainstream mental health community.

For maximum individual benefit, various methodologies of natural healing practices can be used to suit individual differences. Typically, natural healing methods can include (1) traditional meditation—sitting and contemplating; (2) muscle relaxation—moving different groups of body muscles, tensing and releasing to feel the difference; (3) music therapy—listening to soft and soothing music to enter a world of peace; and (4) guided imagery—being guided into a world of creativity to experience the world from a different perspective.

Combining these four types of natural healing methods, this part provides a variety of relaxation, body-mind connection, visual focus, and body-imagery exercises. These exercises aim to encourage clients to use their senses to hear, visualize, breathe, touch, and experientially feel the importance of their existence. This experience should be designed to fit clients' personal needs and characteristics. It is also vital to consult with the client's medical doctor to make sure that this is an appropriate exercise to meet the client's needs.

In guided imagery, as in meditation, concentration and awareness are two essential components in the clinical process. Some clients may enter deep relaxation by focusing their attention on a repeated stimulus or mantra, such as a word (e.g., wonderful, good), a phrase (you are relaxed, you feel great), or a series of actions (breathe in and out, hold your breath and breathe out your troubles). Others benefit more when they are instructed to exercise their mind and find ways to move beyond simple relaxation (Imagine that you are walking through a forest. What do you see? How do you feel as you are approaching a path, a tree, an animal, many trees, many animals?). Instead of inducing sleepiness and disengagement, these exercises intend to engage the mind, while simultaneously creating a suitable environment for relaxation. A quiet environment is helpful, especially during the first few practice sessions, but it is not always a requirement. Tools to assist in meditation are usually kept to a minimum.

Olness and Kohen (1996) divide guided imagery techniques into eight categories: visual imagery, auditory imagery, movement imagery, storytelling, ideomotor, progressive relaxation, eye fixation, and biofeedback. Although eye fixation and biofeedback are not included in this book, the following imagery metaphors have been suggested in the literature in a variety of imagery scripts. These suggestions can help practitioners assist their clients in modifying the guided imagery contents.

1. Visual imagery: favorite places, multiple animals, flower gardens, favorite activities, cloud and sky gazing, color creation and mixture, number counting, alphabet forming, letter writing

2. Auditory imagery: singing a favorite song, playing a musical instrument, listening to music, composing a song, self-talking, talking with an audience

3. Movement imagery: flying blanket, sports activities, bouncing ball, playground activities, walking on a path, planting a tree, floating on a cloud

4. Storytelling: places—path, meadow, river, warm sun, beach, safe place, secluded island; persons—self, parents, siblings, teachers, God, angel, friends, cousins, grandparents, movie stars, singers, prince and princess, queen and king, babies, little boys and girls; animals—rabbit, monkey, cheetah, cat, dog, parrot, bird; others—rainbow, four seasons, leaves, breeze, comfortable feelings, positive outcomes

5. Ideomotor: hold the fists, stretch the arms, relax the muscles, move the body

6. Progressive relaxation: balancing sixteen muscle groups, breathing exercises, giving praise and imagery rewards, relaxing the teddy bear, comparing and contrasting different relaxation stages

Applications

Regular use of relaxation exercises helps clients restore peaceful energy within their bodies and minds. Practical applications are included for each of the guided imagery exercises. The intent of these exercises is to help clients find deeper meaning and insight in their lives and their personal relationships, both within the confines of the therapeutic relationship and on their own. While some of the scripts have a specific treatment focus, others are more general, with the focus evident only in the application and process questions at the end of the exercise. Therapists should feel free to encourage clients to use these more general exercises whenever they feel overwhelmed or stressed, so that they may develop a self-directed relaxation technique. To promote home usage, the therapist can prerecord a tape. Before recommending independent use, however, the therapist should guide the practice of these exercises, so that clients' reactions can be clinically observed and evaluated. In addition, tapes for home usage should include professional instructions, either recorded or prepared in a written format. These instructions are included in the introduction for each exercise in this book.

Guided imagery can be very intense for clients, and clinicians must use sound clinical judgment in using these exercises. The clinician should be mindful that guided imagery is not always appropriate or desirable for every client. Its suitability should be evaluated by assessing the background and mental status of the client, and any religious preferences that may prohibit fanciful imagination. Professionals should be cautious when working with anyone who has had negative experiences with elements related to the imagery, as well as with clients experiencing active hallucinations and those with phobias. The selection of an imagery component (e.g., hill, river, beach, treasure) should be clinically assessed prior to usage of any guided imagery. If appropriate, the clinician can modify the imagery in the exercises to suit individual needs and preferences, and thus avoid any imagery that may be unpleasant or stressful. For clients who have religious preferences that prohibit fanciful imagination or visiting imaginary places, the clinician might modify the exercise or omit guided imagery from therapeutic activities. Being aware of a client's religious preference may also help the clinician adjust exercises to better benefit the client; for example, substituting meaningful religious figures in the guided imagery can help clients feel safe while resolving personal issues.

Even if clients desire to participate in guided imagery, some individuals have difficulty engaging the process. The clinician should use exercise B1, A Preparation Journey, to ascertain the readiness and receptivity of the client in using guided imagery techniques. As with the therapeutic games, careful selection of exercises, ongoing monitoring, and evaluation of outcomes are highly recommended.

Table 3 cross-references the treatment focus of the guided imagery exercises with four broad functions: concentration and awareness, visualization of success, controlling anxiety, and gaining insight. Therapists may use this table as a guide; however, as with the therapeutic games, they should not feel limited by it. Many of the guided imagery scripts can be modified to suit client needs and preferences. For example, an exercise designed for individuals can be used in a group setting where each client is working through individual issues that require a time to relax without group involvement. Likewise, an exercise designed for groups and families can be recorded to be an individual homework assignment.

Suggested Modifications

Since many guided imagery exercises contain complex visualizations that may incite a variety of emotions in clients, take extreme care in choosing an exer-

Table 3 Guided imagery by function and treatment focus

	Function				
	Concentration/ awareness	Visualization of success	Controlling anxiety	Gaining insight	Treatment focus
B1	✓				Suitability assessment
B2		✓	✓	✓	Social inhibition
B3	✓		✓		Learning anxiety
B4	✓	✓			ADHD
B5			✓		Exposure to chronic violence
B6			✓		Medical procedures, pain management
B7	✓				Trauma, social withdrawal, grief
B8			✓		Math anxiety
B9		✓	✓		Teenage fatherhood, affirmation
B10	✓			✓	Abusive parents
B11		✓	✓		Separation anxiety
B12		✓	✓		Test anxiety
B13	✓				Trauma, family violence
B14				✓	Anger control
B15		✓		✓	Self-esteem, daily affirmations, body image
B16			✓		Positive reinforcement
B17				✓	Powerlessness, self-esteem
B18	✓				Grief resolution
B19	✓				Concentration
B20			✓	✓	Anxiety, parent-child conflict
B21				✓	Parent-child relationship
B22	✓				Contrast feelings, anger control
B23	✓				Family, conflict, spirituality

Table 3 (continued) **Guided imagery by function and treatment focus**

	Function			
	Concentration/ awareness	Visualization of success	Controlling anxiety	Gaining insight	Treatment focus
B24	✓				Health restoration
B25				✓	Mental stability
B26		✓		✓	Inner strength, problem solving, anger, family violence, substance abuse
B27			✓		Chronic health issues, depression
B28				✓	Spiritual development
B29				✓	Free association, unconscious reflection
B30				✓	Safety, security

cise. After careful consideration, as presented above, you should be flexible and creative in modifying the imagery. Here are some examples.

1. Use different imagery.

   - For beach or wilderness scenes (B5, B6, B12, B16), substitute soothing urban scenes, watching the sun rise over buildings, city parks, the sound of a train in the distance. This may be especially helpful for those with little experience outside of urban areas.

   - Use imagery that is meaningful to the client. Before starting a guided exercise, ask clients about places they have visited that have been especially soothing and relaxing. Substitute this scene in the imagery.

   - Use music instead of a place; ask clients to think of the "title of a song that you like" or "song lyrics that touch your heart," or to "imagine that you are singing a song you like."

2. Use experts' suggestions (as in the table of suggestions from Olness and Kohen, 1996) to substitute the imagery or change the method of relaxation.

   - Change the imagery within the same type of imagery method:

change "flying on a magic blanket" as a movement to "walking on a path" if the client is height phobic.

- Change the content to another type of imagery: change "visiting a favorable place" (visual) to "composing a song" (auditory).

3. Modify an exercise that focuses on a different therapeutic issue than the one indicated.

- Try "Adolescents Who Are Anxious" (B2) with those who are experiencing performance anxiety in the workplace or at school.

- Try "Children and Adolescents Exposed to Chronic Violence" (B5) with children in crowded or transient living conditions.

4. Ask therapeutic questions from a different imagery exercise to achieve the desired therapeutic purpose.

- Use the questions from "Magic Carpet Ride" (B20) for "Your Place" (B30), and vice versa.

- Try the questions for "Math Anxiety Is Gone!" (B8) with "Dealing with Learning Anxiety" (B3).

Guided Imagery for Children and Adolescents

B1
A Preparation Journey
Monit Cheung

This exercise is based on Olness and Kohen's suggestion of ideomotor techniques (1996), and Hunter's basic induction technique (1994). It helps clients realize the importance of concentration. It is also a good assessment tool to determine whether an individual client is a good candidate for guided imagery exercises or other hypnotherapeutic applications. During the exercise, if the client's right hand drifts downward, this client may benefit from a variety of relaxation and guided imagery exercises.

Script

Stand up, please. Distance your feet shoulder-length apart so that your body can have better support.

Relax. Take a deep breath. Stretch both arms out straight in front of you with the palms of your hands facing up. Right. Relax. Now close your eyes. Imagine that I am putting a book on your right palm. This is a book you'd like to read. You notice that your right arm begins to feel pretty heavy, but you say in your mind, "It's OK." [Pause.] Now imagine that a second book is placed on top of the first book. It's heavy. Your right arm can really feel the heaviness, and it wants to drift down. Let it drift down a little. Good! It's getting even heavier. Now imagine that I am placing a third book on top. You think that these books are interesting, but they are very heavy. In your mind now, relax and let your right hand drift downward. The books feel heavier and heavier. Your right hand is moving down more and more. Good! It's just the way it should be. You are doing a great job. Don't move your hands when you are ready to open your eyes. Keep them the way they are. Now open your eyes and see your hands.

Application

Although this exercise is an assessment tool, it can also be used as a short exercise to help clients concentrate and recognize the interaction between their mind and body. It is important not to impose any suggestive comments during this exercise, such as a problem the client may have encountered. After the exercise is over, have clients do some gentle body movements, such as stretching their arms and legs and taking three deep breaths. They can then discuss how they felt before, during, and after this exercise.

B2

Adolescents Who Are Anxious

Mark F. Akerlund

This exercise was created for adolescents who experience anxiety in social situations or have difficulty in communicating and expressing themselves. Its purpose is to enable clients to identify how negative thoughts influence their feelings and behavior. With its cognitive-behavioral nature, clients learn how to identify physical stress in their bodies. Through this exercise, clients teach themselves to recognize the relationship between physical and emotional tension. This exercise helps clients challenge irrational beliefs while simultaneously learning how to relax.

Script

Make sure that you are comfortable. Sit in a chair or lie down. Do whatever you need to do in order to enhance this time that you have set aside for yourself. Begin by dimming the lights and taking a deep breath, breathing in through your nose and out through your mouth. Breathe deeply and slowly. As you breathe, you are relaxing your body and mind. As you exhale, you are releasing stress, tension, and anxiety. Continue breathing deeply and slowly and tell yourself how you feel in your mind.

My hands are heavy. My hands are warm. My hands are heavy and warm.

My arms are heavy. My arms are warm. My arms are heavy and warm.

My shoulders are heavy . . . my shoulders are warm . . . my shoulders are heavy and warm. I am relaxed

My legs are heavy . . . my legs are warm . . . my legs are heavy and warm.

My feet are heavy . . . my feet are warm . . . my feet are heavy and warm.

I am at peace with myself . . . I am safe . . . I am relaxed.

Feel the relaxation spread from your shoulders down to your arms, to your hands. Feel the tension leave your body like drops of water dripping off your fingertips. [Pause.]

Now take a moment to identify a social situation where you feel stress, tension, or anxiety. Play the scene in your mind. [Pause for ten seconds.] Now remove this scene from your mind and relax. Imagine the scene again. This time you feel confident, relaxed, and in control . . . Re-create the scene in your mind . . . with a positive outcome. I am confident . . . I am relaxed . . . I am in control . . . I choose what is best for me. Notice how your positive thoughts make you feel positive . . . make you feel relaxed in all situations. Take a few moments to enjoy your relaxation . . . let your mind wander. [Repeat exercise several times.] Let your mind take you to a place where you feel warm, confident, and safe . . . When you're ready, count backward from ten and slowly open your eyes. 10, 9, 8, 7, 6, 5, 4, 3, 2, 1. Open your eyes and look around. You are safe and relaxed.

Application

Relaxation training and guided imagery should be followed by cognitive-behavioral therapy in order to reinforce the benefits of positive thinking and challenge irrational beliefs, as well as to reframe clients' belief system as it interferes with social functioning. Therapeutic questions can include

1. Name a situation that can cause anxiety, stress, or tension.
2. Have you experienced this situation in the past?
3. How do you usually feel when you experience anxiety, stress, or tension?
4. During this exercise, what situation reminded you of anxiety? What came to your mind?
5. When you were asked during this exercise to replace tension with relaxation, how did you feel? What did you do to make the shift?
6. When you managed to make a shift from being anxious to feeling confident, what came to your mind?
7. What was in the newly created scene that helped you relax?
8. Could you name additional elements in this scene that could be used in the future to think about relaxation?

B3

Dealing with Learning Anxiety

Sharon Clark Peska and Monit Cheung

This relaxation script can be prerecorded with a musical background. The tape may be used once a day for fifteen minutes. It helps children and adolescents when they become anxious or are unable to concentrate in school or at home. Initially, it is recommended that a parent participate with the child to ensure that the child understands the purpose of the exercise and does it properly.

Begin by showing the child pictures of wonderful places, clipped from travel magazines. Permit the child to choose a picture he or she likes, and then instruct the child to sit or lie in a comfortable position in a quiet room. Dim the lights and turn on the tape recorder.

Script

Hello. It's time to take a trip to a wonderful place. First, make yourself comfortable. Stretch out and let your body relax. Now close your eyes and relax. Make a fist with both hands. Are you feeling tense? Let your hands relax and feel the relaxation. Check your shoulders; is there any tension? Let it all go. Think about your forehead, take a deep breath, and let go of all the tension. Think about your stomach, your muscles, your body . . . let all tensions go, and relax. Now concentrate on your legs. Relax and think, "I feel good." Take a deep breath and think, "I feel wonderful!" Say it again in your mind, "I feel wonderful!" Take another deep breath, and think one more time, "I feel wonderful!" [Pause.] With each breath, you feel more and more relaxed and wonderful. It's such a wonderful feeling to be relaxed.

Let's take a trip to the place that you chose. Enjoy this wonderful place. It's a beautiful day. The sky is blue, and this place is quiet and peaceful. You are walking on a path. This path is so soft, so comfortable. This is a path leading you to a wonderful land. You said to yourself, "I feel wonderful!"

Imagine that you see a friend coming toward you. This is a friend that you like, but you do not want this friend to be here now. You want to be alone. You want to shout, "Go away," but your friend smiles. You like this smile very much. It reminds you of a wonderful person you know. Your friend says, "How are you?" You feel so relaxed that you did not tell this friend to go away. You feel all your tensions disappear. You feel so relaxed. Take a deep breath, say it in your heart, "I feel wonderful! I feel wonderful!"

You continue your walk into this place. You like this place and want to stay longer. You see your teacher coming toward you. You don't want to go. You want to shout, "Go away," but your teacher smiles. You like this smile very much. It reminds you of a wonderful person you know. Your teacher says, "How are you?" You tell your teacher politely, "I want to stay longer; may I?" You feel so relaxed that you did not tell your teacher to go away. All your tensions disappear. You feel so relaxed. Take a deep breath, say it in your heart, "I feel wonderful! I feel wonderful!"

Think about this wonderful place you like. Let all the tensions go. Relax your body, take a deep breath, and tell yourself, "I feel wonderful! I feel wonderful!"

Now you are leaving this place and going to school. You are sitting at your desk at school. Imagine that you are taking a test and having trouble remembering an answer. You tell yourself, "Don't worry! I can manage." Now take a deep breath, relax, and you will find it easier to recall your memory. Yes, you can do it! You say to yourself, "Yes, I can do it! I feel wonderful! I feel wonderful!" Anytime when you find it difficult, or when you feel anxious, remember to take a deep breath and relax. You can do it!

This wonderful feeling is with you always. You want to be yourself and feel relaxed. Come back and visit. Keep your eyes closed for a few more minutes and say to yourself, "Tomorrow will be a better day than today because I am learning how to be relaxed. Whenever I have a problem, I will relax and find the answer for it."

Now open your eyes. Listen to the music for a few minutes. When it is finished, you may return to your studies or play, or if you are ready for bed, you may drift off to sleep. I'll talk with you again later. [Music continues to play.]

Application

After practicing this exercise with the child, encourage the child to write down "I feel wonderful," "Don't worry! I can manage," and "Yes, I can do it" as his or her affirmation statements. Introduce the tape to the parent and instruct the parent to observe the child while the child is listening to the tape at home. When the child appears to be restless or emotionally upset, the parent can encourage the child to listen to the tape. The parent should check if the child's eyes and forehead are relaxed before, during, and after the relaxation exercise. After the exercise, the parent or therapist can ask how the child is feeling at that moment. The adult should then record the child's response on a scale from 1 to 5, with 1 being extremely relaxed and 5 being extremely tense. This will help the child, the parent(s), and the therapist to monitor the child's progress.

ADHD Kids

Monit Cheung

Children with attention deficit or hyperactivity disorder (ADHD) usually have difficulty remaining seated when required to do so. They tend to talk excessively, interrupt others, and do not seem to be able to sustain attention in class or play activities. They often do not listen to what is being said. Therefore, it is very important to provide them with some hints regarding their limitations so that they learn to concentrate. Biofeedback and relaxation have been proven to be effective in treating ADHD children, not only by reducing their stress and anxiety, but also by increasing their skills in following clues (Finley & Jones, 1992; Monastra, 2005). This exercise is short, as it is aimed at helping children who have a short attention span.

Script

This is a relaxation exercise for you. Now close your eyes and stretch your arms and legs. Take a really deep breath and settle down comfortably. When you hear the number one, you will take a deep breath again, exhale, and feel the relaxation. Let's practice it . . . *one*—take a deep breath, exhale, and feel the relaxation. Very good!

Paying attention is difficult, isn't it? Not anymore! You can do it. Just remember *one*, then take a deep breath and relax. Excellent!

Talking with other kids in your class when your teacher asks you not to? Not anymore! You can avoid it. Just remember *one*—take a deep breath and relax. Yes, it is the way to do it. You can do it.

Sometimes you can't settle down? Not anymore! You can settle down very quickly by remembering *one*—breathe in, hold it, and out. Feel how relaxed you are. Say it in your mind, "Yes, I can relax!"

Whenever you feel like talking or getting into other people's activities, just remember *one*. Yes, it is simple. Say in your mind, "I can do it."

It is great that you can concentrate and relax. I am going to count backward from five to one. When you hear *one*, you know what to do, right?

5 . . . 4 . . . 3 . . . 2 . . . now open your eyes . . . *one*.

Application

It is important to help ADHD children learn how to relax and concentrate. This short relaxation routine can be used as a beginning ritual every time the child is seen. In subsequent sessions, guide the child to add other kinds of learning to the list, such as *two,* representing "I can concentrate!" or simply "Concentrate!"; and *three,* representing "I can stop and think" or simply "Stop and think!"

It is recommended that this list not be too long. If the child wants to include more than two clues, do one exercise with two clues at the beginning of the session and the other exercise with additional clues at the end. If children contribute to their own lists, they will be more likely to use the clues in their daily activities to remind themselves to relax. After they master the first clue, encourage children to ask their parents to use their clues (one, two, three, etc.) to remind them when they do not seem to be concentrating. This will empower the children to take charge of their situation.

B5

Children and Adolescents Exposed to Chronic Violence

Tracy A. Middleton

This exercise is designed to induce relaxation in children and adolescents who have been exposed to chronic violence, especially in witnessing violence in the inner city. These children are often anxious and live in persistent states of fear, resulting in physiological hyperarousal and hyperactivity. The progressive muscle relaxation in this exercise counters the physiological hyperarousal, and the images that are generated evoke a sense of peace, security, and safety.

Script

Find a comfortable position, either sitting in a chair or lying on the floor. Close your eyes. Breathe slowly and deeply: inhale . . . exhale . . . inhale . . . exhale. As you exhale, feel the release of pressure . . . relax . . . release the tension in your body.

Notice your right arm, paying attention to your right fist. Clench it tightly. Feel the tension in your hand and forearm. [Pause.] Now release. Relax the right hand and release the tension. Notice the difference between tension and re- laxation. [Pause.] Now let's do the same with the left hand. Clench your left fist tightly. Feel the tension in your hand and forearm. [Pause.] Now release. Relax the left hand and release the tension. Notice the difference between tension and relaxation. [Pause.] Now tighten both hands into fists and pull them in toward your shoulders. Tighten the muscles in your upper arms. Feel the tension . . . relax. Let your arms fall to your sides. Feel the difference between tension and release.

Now the shoulders. Pull your shoulders up toward your ears. Hold them there and feel the tension. Now relax. [Pause.] Now let's work on the neck muscles. Press your head against the back of your chair or the floor. Notice any tension in the back of your neck and upper back. Hold the tension. [Pause.] Release and relax.

Move your relaxation down to your stomach. Tighten your abdominal muscles. Hold it. [Pause.] Now relax. Let your muscles feel totally loose. [Pause.] Now let's focus on the legs. Squeeze your thigh muscles. Tighten. [Pause.] Now re- lease. Feel the difference. Now the lower legs. Pretend a string is pulling your toes toward the ceiling. Tighten the calf muscles. Feel the pulling sensation. [Pause.] Now release.

Allow your legs to feel totally relaxed. Now scan your body for any remaining tension. Relax your arms. Release the tension. Let go of the pressure in your shoulders. Relax all the muscles of your stomach and your back. Let the tension drain from your thighs, legs, feet, and toes. Allow all the muscles of your body to relax. Remain quiet. Keep your eyes closed and feel the relaxation.

Allow yourself to be taken away. You are now seeing a beautiful ocean beach. The sky is clear and blue, and the sun is bright and warm. A gentle breeze caresses your cheek. Inhale the air. The smell of ocean salt surrounds you. It's fresh and clean. Drifting above you is a perfectly formed cloud that reminds you of a soft pillow. You feel safe . . . peaceful . . . and calm. You walk slowly along the shore of the beautiful beach with its white sands and clear, blue water. The warm water brushes against your bare feet, leaving a trace of foam as it passes. As you walk, the sun warms your neck and back . . . the warmth spreads throughout your body. You feel totally relaxed and calm. You take a few moments to enjoy this feeling.

Listen to the sounds around you. You hear the sound of the waves coming in. Birds are flying above. A seagull spreads its wings and flies above you while other birds sing in the distance. You walk farther. Feel the soft, white sand slip between your toes. It's a beautiful day. You notice a large palm tree, and you sit in the shade of its leaves. The sweet aroma of gardenias surrounds you. Feelings of comfort, peace, and safety are within you. Experience this moment fully. You experience more comfort with each moment you spend in this peaceful place. Every part of your body is feeling total peace and comfort. Feel the comfort in your arms . . . it moves slowly to your neck and back, like the waves in front of you. The sensation moves to your shoulders . . . Enjoy this feeling. Let your muscles rest . . . Send the message of relaxation to every part of your body.

This is your place . . . you can visit it anytime you want. It's so beautiful and peaceful. You are happy and safe.

Now begin to take deeper breaths. I will count backward from five. Upon hearing the number 1, you will open your eyes feeling alert and relaxed. 5, 4, 3, 2, 1.

Application

After the exercise, process the client's feelings and find concrete suggestions to deal with difficult feelings associated with the identified problem.

1. What feelings did you have before starting this exercise?
2. What feelings did you have while hearing me count backward from five to one?

3. How might this exercise help you when you are stressed?
4. In what situations might this exercise be helpful?
5. What images can you think of when you want to relax?
6. Tell me your definitions of peace (security, safety, justice, etc.).
7. Within your definitions, what elements are the most important to help you relax?

Medical Procedures
Renata Domatti

This script was created for children and adolescents who must undergo painful medical procedures or who are facing a terminal illness. This exercise helps clients relax and focus their attention on something other than the current situation. This allows the doctor to complete the medical procedure quickly and lessens the discomfort for the patient. By focusing and relaxing, children may more easily discuss their feelings and fears about death and dying.

A beach scene is used in this example, but allow the child to determine the scene where the guided imagery will take place. It is important to allow the client to select the scenario and actively participate in order to maximize a sense of control.

This script can be prerecorded on an audiotape. Speak slowly, in a soft, soothing tone. The tape should not exceed more than a few minutes, as most medical procedures are relatively short.

Script

[Appropriate music can be played in the background to help relaxation.]

Begin by closing your eyes and taking a deep breath. Imagine a place you would like to be at this moment, for instance, the beach.

You step out onto the sand. It's a soft beige color and it is warm on your bare feet. The sand moves between your toes as you walk toward the water. You can feel the cool breeze and the warm sun against your face. You're already feeling much more relaxed. You look up and see a brightly colored kite with a long tail flying in the sky. It glides up and down in a very soft motion. Along with the kite, there are several seagulls. They are flying and diving toward the water. They look so free and peaceful. You take some bread out of your pocket. You have been saving it for this moment. You throw a handful into the air and watch the seagulls dive above your head to grab the bread. Some of the bread drops at your feet, and the seagulls land near you and pick at it.

You walk to the edge of the water. The water rushes up over your toes and covers your feet. The water is cool and soothing. You turn and see several children playing in the sand. You watch for a moment as they build a small sand castle. They are trying so hard to make it stay together that they don't notice you. Their castle is crumbling, but they don't give up. They keep adding more sand and more water. You sense deep willpower in them.

You turn back to the water. It is icy blue today. The waves are high. You watch as each wave swells, crashes into the water, and then rushes toward your feet. The timing is perfect. One wave then another, then another, then another, and another. It's mesmerizing. You can't turn your eyes away. It's so relaxing. So you take a few steps back and sit in the sand. You watch as each wave swells and crashes rhythmically into the water.

[Sounds of waves crashing follow the script.]

Application

Discuss the medical procedures with the client. If possible, talk with the client before and after each procedure. Try to probe the client's feelings of pain and the effectiveness of the guided imagery for pain management. If face-to-face interactions are not feasible, have the client keep a journal of each medical procedure that can be used during discussion at a later time. It is also important to work with hospital staff such as nurses, doctors, and child life specialists to further understand the client's feelings. Here are sample questions that can be used during discussion.

1. List or describe the feelings that you experienced during the medical procedure.
2. Were the feelings overwhelming?
3. Did the tape help you relax? What else might help you relax?
4. What positive images can you use to minimize your pain?
5. What did you learn in this exercise that can be taught to other children in this situation/hospital?

B7

Traumatized Children

Colleen Knox

Use this exercise with children who are inhibited and unable to express joy, creativity, or imaginative play owing to trauma or a temperamental tendency to protect themselves through withdrawal. The process begins with a relaxation component in hopes of helping the children to be open to the experience and to whatever feelings emerge.

Before beginning this exercise, make sure that the child does not have a fear of heights.

Script

Lie back. Get very comfortable, with your hands by your side. Close your eyes and concentrate on your breathing. Take nice, deep, long breaths. Feel the air moving gently in and out of your lungs. Breathe in and out; and in and out. You're feeling very relaxed. [Pause.]

Imagine that you are lying on a grassy slope. The grass is thick and feels wonderfully soft. It is a beautiful, sunny day with a slightly cool breeze to keep you comfortable. As you look up at the sky, you notice the vivid blue background behind the large, white, fluffy clouds. All your muscles are relaxed, and as you relax, your body begins to feel lighter.

Against the background of the blue sky and white clouds, you notice several scissortail birds sweeping back and forth through the sky. You admire their long tails and gracefulness.

You feel the warmth of the sun intensify, and the breeze flowing over you getting stronger. You see another flock of smaller birds. They appear and disappear as they circle in and out of the large white clouds. As you watch the birds, you marvel at the ease of their flight and at their playful freedom as they traverse the sky.

You feel completely in control of your actions as you begin to glide into the sky. You feel the rush of wind on your face. You decide to join in the game of hide-and-seek with the birds. It is a wonderful feeling to fly and join the other birds. You watch as several birds enter the clouds, and you wonder what it is like inside the cloud.

Entering the cloud, you expect to see nothing but white. Instead, you find yourself surrounded by a beautiful spray of light. You are surprised to be entering this beautiful sight. Lights dance off glistening drops of water, making colorful rainbows in every direction. The water drops from the cloud soothe your body from the increased warmth of the sun. The drops begin to build on your skin, developing into droplets. First, there are hundreds, then thousands, getting larger and larger until they finally drip off your body. The drips tickle as they travel along your body, and you laugh from the feeling. You can even feel the change of temperature as you enter and exit the cloud. The sun's warm rays are followed by the coolness inside the cloud.

Now the sky is beginning to turn orange, and the sun will soon set. As the rich green of the forest turns darker, you are surprised to see lights in the distance. Instead of circling back up toward the sky with the other birds, you are curious and want to see where the lights are coming from. Flying rapidly toward the lights, you notice that they seem to disappear as you get close to them, yet you see more in the distance. Each time you get close to one, it disappears! You decide to slow down and see if the lights continue to disappear.

As you slow, you notice a firefly flying right beside you and glowing brightly. Its color is soft green. Then it is gone. The darkness is replaced by other lights of various colors, blinking on and off all around you. Hundreds of fireflies surround you, all of them blinking on and off. It's like a fairyland of lights, and you feel as though you are in a magical land. You gently land on the forest floor, relaxed and excited from your play with the birds. Walking slowly through the forest, you feel the moss of the forest floor on your bare feet. It feels soft and cool.

As you continue on your way, you see a house ahead of you. Its lights are on and it looks welcoming. The house seems familiar, like you've been here before and it was a nice place to be. It feels like a safe place to spend the night. You enter and find a bowl of your favorite warm food. Being very hungry from your afternoon of fun, you enjoy the meal, which fills your belly. Now feeling very content, you wander through the house and find a soft, comfortable place to lie down. Pulling the blanket up over your body, you fall fast asleep. When you awaken, you will feel refreshed and happy.

What you've just experienced was an imaginary place to relax you, to take you away from any discomfort, and to make you feel happy. It is now time to come back to reality to talk. Are you ready? Stretch . . . wiggle your fingers and toes . . . open your eyes and return to this room.

Application

Process some feeling questions after the exercise.

1. What feelings did you have as you watched the birds? Flew through the sky? Walked through the forest?
2. We sometimes have some bad feelings that we dislike. What kind of

bad feelings would you like to leave behind? What would you suggest to children of your age to do to get rid of these bad feelings?

3. What feelings from this exercise do you want to keep with you today? How will you keep those feelings?

4. What would you say or do when you feel happy? What would you suggest to children of your age to say or do in order to feel happier?

Math Anxiety Is Gone!

Patrick Leung

Teaching mathematics requires patience, understanding, and the ability to explain in a step-by-step manner. Unfortunately, many children and adults who went through the process of learning did not have teachers with these essential qualities. Helping children and older students deal with math anxiety has become an important task for many schoolteachers, counselors, and parents.

This relaxation exercise encourages the use of all five senses to welcome numbers. It is a systematic desensitization technique to help students overcome math phobias and to learn to love numbers.

Script

Hello, this is a trip to a beautiful garden. Let's relax and think about a fruit you would like to grow and eat. What is it? An apple? A pear? A cherry? Oh yes, you find what you like. What color is it? How many colors does it have? One, two, or three? Does it have seeds? How many seeds do you see? A few or many? It is certainly a very tasty fruit. Is it cool and crispy, or is it warm and soft? Imagine you are growing your fruit in this beautiful garden. You put in some seeds, 1, 2, 3, 4, 5 . . . You are counting the seeds as you plant them in the soil. That's beautiful! You love it.

You keep watering your seeds. You like this garden very much. You are watching the plants grow. How many plants do you have? 1, 2, 3, 4, 5 . . . You are counting the plants as they come out from the soil one by one. One plus one equals two. Three plus one plus one equals five. That's beautiful! You love it.

You keep watching your plants grow. You are lying down on the grass and watching the clouds. You feel the warm sun and see the clouds slowly approaching you. The clouds are changing colors. They are white, yellow, orange, pink, purple, green . . . How pretty they are! That's beautiful! You love it.

You keep watching the clouds. The clouds change into different shapes and numbers. They are soft and fun. They are chasing each other. One times one equals one. All the ones are chasing each other and having fun. Two times nine equals eighteen. 10, 20, 30, 40, 50, 60, 70, 80, 90, 100—these numbers look very friendly. You love to watch them.

You are relaxed. You smell the sweetness of your fruit. You love it. It reminds you of the numbers you just saw. It is as sweet as ten, as beautiful as twenty, as wonderful as one hundred, and you love to think about them. 5, 10, 15, 20, 25, 30, 35, 40, 45, 50, you love to count them. 55, 60, 65, 70, 75, 80, 85, 90, 95, 100, you finish counting and you are very relaxed.

You are very happy. You eat your fruit. You eat 1, 2, 3, 4, 5 . . . You love them. You find a small stick and begin writing numbers on the sand. You are counting how many plants you had, how many fruits you ate, how many clouds you saw, how many numbers you counted—these are good memories. You love to think about them.

You are about to leave this beautiful garden. You love the numbers you saw, you love the numbers you counted, you love the shapes of these numbers. You are going to think about doing math at home. You will relax when you see these numbers. You will do your math with patience, just like what you did with your plants. You will do your math with understanding, just like what you did with your clouds. You will do your math with detailed explanations, just like what you did with counting.

Relax and take a deep breath. Slowly breathe in, 1, 2, 3 . . . Slowly breathe out, 3, 2, 1. Tell yourself, "I can do it!"

When I count from one to ten, you will feel refreshed and ready to do your work. [Slowly counting] 1, 2, 3, 4, 5, 6, 7, 8, 9, 10. Have confidence in yourself and have a nice day.

Application

This exercise is designed for people of all age groups who want to relax. It is not limited to people with math anxiety. The simple math in the script may be replaced with something more difficult (e.g., algebra or statistical formulas) for students who are experiencing difficulties with advanced math or statistics. In order to therapeutically help children express difficulties experienced at school or school phobias, help them relax first and then follow up with questions to process their feelings.

1. What came to your mind when you felt relaxed?

2. When numbers are counted in this exercise, what did you think about? Re-count from one to ten slowly [counting]; now tell me what is the meaning of each number? What is one? Two? Which number do you like? Dislike?

3. Tell me what you like about school. What do you dislike?

Parenting for Teenage Fathers
Ed Muldrow

This script was created for teenage fathers for the improvement of problem solving, decision making, and parenting skills. This exercise helps teenage fathers use visualization in coping with the problems of adolescent parenthood. The imagery combined with the brief relaxation section can help a father recognize his feelings, and it is hoped that it can increase home use of guided imagery and visualization. Visualization can offer an important step in forming a clear mental picture of oneself, and it can encourage performance based on the most positive vision in a variety of situations.

Script

Hello. Congratulate yourself for taking an important step into your future by participating in this guided imagery exercise, *Parenting for Teenage Fathers.* In listening to this, you are making a commitment to improve your skills in coping with the problems and stresses that new fathers often experience. Notice that you can and will remain aware at all times while listening to this, and you can easily respond to any emergency in an appropriate manner.

Let's begin by sitting or lying down in a relaxed position. Become aware of your goal to improve your skills in coping with the problems you experience as a teenage father. Close your eyes. Let yourself become aware of a small problem or stressful event that has occurred recently in your experience as a father. Let yourself think about it for a few seconds. [Pause.] As you are thinking about this problem or event, notice which places in your body feel tension. Now let those body muscles and tensions tighten. Tighten those muscles and let them become very tense. Hold this tightness, and count from one to ten. Now relax [pause] and let go. [Pause.] As you relax your muscles, notice the difference between tensing your muscles and relaxing them. Take a deep, round, belly breath. Let go as you continue to relax and breathe from your belly. Feel your chest expand.

One way to cope with the stresses of parenting is to get in touch with your body, to feel the tensions of tightening muscles and then to let them go. As you let go, notice if any helpful idea, thought, sound, or solution moves into your awareness. It may be something that you have not thought about before, or it may be something that you know for sure. Now remember what caused the problem or stressful event you were thinking of before, and notice that it is less powerful now, that it is not affecting you now. It has moved away in the distance, farther away.

Now take another deep, belly breath. Relax and let go. Enjoy the calm and peaceful feeling that comes with taking the time to do something beneficial for yourself. Now think of an experience you had as a father that resulted in frustration. Think about your actions in that situation. At what point did you begin to feel frustrated? What was the outcome of the situation? Now visualize yourself in that situation being powerful, yet calm and relaxed. What would you do differently to cope with the frustration? What would others do? Now with a relaxed feeling, visualize yourself changing the outcome, so it is exactly the way you want it. What would you be feeling? Experience the feelings of relaxation and success.

Now imagine you are writing a note to yourself or to another person, in order to share the problems and stresses you have experienced as a father. Start the note with "Dear . . ." Now think deeply about what you will write. [Pause five seconds.] Imagine you write down all the problems you have had and all stressful events that have occurred. [Pause.] Now imagine that you take that note, with all those frustrated feelings written on it, and set it aside for twenty-four hours. Just put it away. Allow some time to let the problems and stresses go. Visualize yourself waving good-bye to all those problems. Now imagine that you are sharing your problems and stresses with someone you trust. Say it in your mind, "I am frustrated but I can cope with it. I need a listener." Feel how good it is to be able to tell someone about the problems and stresses that come with parenting and being a teenage father. Now take another deep, belly breath. Relax and let go.

I will now count to five. At five, you will open your eyes, feeling a sense of renewed energy, calmness, and strength. 1, 2, 3, 4, 5 . . . Now stretch, take a big stretch, and take a deep, round, belly breath. Have a good one!

Application

As a written assignment after the guided imagery exercise, the adolescent father can design ways to cope with problems and stresses. Suggest that the client write affirmations on a poster board, or ask the client to visualize himself seated at a desk, writing these affirmations in his favorite-color marker on a large white poster board.

1. I have a choice in the way that I cope with the problems and stresses I experience as a father, and I do not have to let problems control me.

2. I have made a choice to cope with problems and stresses in a way that will allow me to have experiences of success and satisfaction both as a person and as a father.

3. Every problem I encounter can show me how to be better prepared in the future.

4. I believe that I will achieve success in improving my problem solving, decision making, and parenting skills.

During group discussions, use the following questions:

1. Are you willing to examine your past, let go of your emotional reactions to these experiences, and make changes in your life for the future?

2. Do you expect the best of yourself?

3. How did you feel after using the guided imagery exercise at home?

Physical Abuse and Role Reversal

Beth Tauber

This exercise was created for parents or caregivers who have physically abused their children. It attempts to help parents involved with the children's protective service to develop empathy for children who have been physically abused. It uses role reversal in which parent participants return to memories of their own childhood, and experience the situations that their children have had while in their care. By feeling the emotional reactions to the abuse, hopefully the parents will develop greater empathy and will work toward finding more appropriate methods for relating to and disciplining their children.

Script

Find a comfortable position. Relax. Close your eyes and become very relaxed. Take a deep breath in. Now let it out. Take another deep breath in. Now let it out. Feel that your head is very relaxed. Feel that your shoulders are relaxed. Your arms are feeling very relaxed. Take another deep breath and relax your chest. Feel your legs begin to relax. Let your knees relax. Finally, allow your feet to relax. Take another deep breath and let it out, feeling that your entire body is relaxed.

Now picture yourself as a young child between six and eight years old. Remember a moment in your young childhood when you are playful, cheerful, and happy. Sit with this child who is enjoying life. Picture what this child is doing. Feel the joy that this child feels while engaging in this activity that brings her pleasure.

Now imagine Lisa is the child, and she is excited and active. Picture Lisa playing and doing the things she enjoys. Now imagine that Lisa suddenly realizes she is late for dinner. Her heart begins to race and beat out of control. Her heart beats so hard she fears it will jump out of her chest. Lisa, once playful and joyful, is suddenly anxious and panicked. She quickly forgets what she has been involved in and races toward home. She feels short of breath, but cannot stop for fear of being even later getting home.

Lisa runs as fast as she can to get home. Suddenly, she trips over a tree branch and falls. She pulls herself up and notices she has splattered mud all over herself. From her fear and exhaustion, she begins to cry, and her precious little body shakes out of control. She finds the energy inside herself to get up and continue running toward home. She runs even harder than she had before.

When Lisa finally reaches her home, she stumbles up the stairs of the porch—out of breath, trying to remain calm. She prays silently to herself that she is not too late getting home. She takes a deep breath before pulling the door open. As she quietly opens the door, so as not to draw attention to herself or disturb anyone, she hears her parents arguing in the next room. She is a bit relieved that maybe she can sneak into her room and change her muddy clothes without anyone noticing. She instantly senses the familiar odor of smoke and beer. She begins to take small steps toward her room, when her mother shouts at her to get into the kitchen. Lisa is startled and jumps. The fear and panic return as she hesitates to move toward the kitchen. As she gains the courage to move into the kitchen, she rounds the corner to approach the door, and her mother catches a glimpse of her. Her mother yells at Lisa for the dirt on her clothing, telling her she does not appreciate what she has, that she is a spoiled brat and cannot take care of anything. Lisa looks down at the floor in shame. She hopes to be sent to her room to change.

Her mother yells at her, "Take those filthy clothes off and sit down now." Lisa tries to ask to go change, but her mother continues to yell at her, "Shut up. You have nothing to say. You are late again. You are so inconsiderate." Lisa sits in the chair quietly, hoping her mother will not make her take off her clothes before dinner. She sits staring down at the floor when all of the sudden, slap. Her mother swings her hand against the child's face. "I told you to take off those filthy clothes."

Tears begin to flow down Lisa's face as she begins to undress. She hesitantly removes the clothes and sits back down. Her mother throws a plate of food in front of her and says, "Here, you brat." Lisa looks down at the food. All of the sudden, Lisa feels the familiar stings on her back as her mother yells and begins striking her with the rope saying, "You can't even say thank you. I told you not to be late. I told you to take care of your things. You are such a brat and do not deserve anything." Lisa tries to make it through, and prays it will soon be over. Her mother finally throws down the rope. Lisa looks at the rope and notices fresh blood splattered on the rope and on the floor. Lisa knows it will be a long night of pain and fear.

Lisa's father stumbles into the kitchen, laughing at the girl who is sitting at the table, freshly beaten and nearly naked. Her father sits at the table. Lisa can feel him mocking her without even looking at him. It is a familiar event in her family. She sits quietly, praying the night will pass quickly and soon she will be safe at school.

Now you will come back to our session. Relax. Take a deep breath and open your eyes as you let it go. Take another deep breath and let it go.

Application

This is a role-reversal technique that places an abusive parent or caretaker in a child's position in order to experience the child's feelings and relive the parent's childhood. After the guided exercise, you can use the following questions to help the parent or caretaker address feelings and thoughts:

1. List the feelings the young child might have experienced.

2. What feelings/reactions do you have after listening to this story?

3. In what ways did the parents react inappropriately to the child?

4. What message would you like to share with other parents?

5. Share with me any other thoughts you might have about your children.

B11
Reducing Separation Anxiety
Demori Currid Driver

This exercise is for children aged four to eight who experience separation anxiety. It can show them how to relax and control anxiety when they are away from their primary caregiver. If the separation anxiety occurs in a day-care or school setting, teachers and other caregivers should be told how to encourage the child to use the exercise.

Script

Find a comfortable place to sit or lie down. We're going to start by taking some deep breaths to relax. Ready? OK, breathe in as much as you can, and breathe out slowly and softly. Good. Let's try it again. Breathe in as much as your lungs will let you, and breathe out slowly and softly. Great. Now close your eyes and do it. Breathe in deeply, and breathe out slowly and softly. Three more. In . . . out . . . good. Again. In . . . out. Last one. In . . . slowly, as deep as you can, and out slowly . . . good job.

OK, keep your eyes closed. In your head, I want you to picture yourself in your classroom at school. Imagine all the other kids there; imagine you can see all their faces. Imagine the room. Think about what the walls look like, what the floor looks like, what the whole room looks like. Imagine your teacher. She is in front of the classroom speaking to the class. It is almost time for you to go home. You know that your mom is waiting for you outside. You are very excited to see her and to tell her about your day. You know that she will hug you and be happy to see you. The bell rings, and your teacher leads you outside. You see your mom standing in her usual spot. She looks so happy to see you! She looks so proud of you for working hard in school all day! Picture her face. See her big smile. Take one of those deep breaths. In . . . out. Good! You feel happy and relaxed.

[For young children or with those who have difficulty sustaining attention, it may be wise to stop at this point and discuss their feelings before continuing.]

OK, now picture yourself in the classroom again. This time picture the room in the morning before school starts. See all the other kids coming in with their backpacks and lunches. Imagine the room. Imagine your teacher. She is getting ready for the day ahead. You know your mom has to leave soon. You feel sad and anxious. Your chest feels tight. You want to cry. You know she has to leave. Can you see her in your head? How do you feel? Now, I want you to take one of those deep breaths. Ready? In . . . out. Good. Now you are going to count to three. Ready, count with me, 1, 2, 3. Now picture your mom's face at the end of the day, her big, happy smile; she is so proud of you for being brave in school all day. Clear your mind of everything but her face. Do you feel the bad feelings going away? OK, let's practice again. It's the beginning of the day, and you know your mom has to leave. Imagine how you are feeling. She is walking out the door. Take one of those deep breaths, count 1, 2, 3, and now picture her happy face at the end of the day. Good. Now imagine it's the middle of the day, and you really start to miss your mom. You feel very sad. Take a deep breath, count 1, 2, 3, and picture her face, so happy to see you at the end of the day. Good! You feel relaxed and happy. You know your mom will be proud of you for being brave. You know you can work and play with all your classmates without feeling sad. You know you can make it through the day.

Anytime you feel like you miss your mom, I want you to close your eyes, take a deep breath, and count to three in your head. After you count to three, I want you to picture your mom's face and how she looks at you at the end of the day—so happy to see you and so proud of you for being brave.

Now we are going to take five more of those deep breaths, and you are going to open your eyes. Ready? In . . . as much as your lungs will let you, and out . . . In . . . and out, slowly and softly. In . . . out. Two more. In . . . and out. Last one. In as deep as you can, and out. Good! Open your eyes.

Application

This exercise is a solutions-based approach for children with a stable caregiver. It is not intended to treat traumatized children or those with attachment disorders. "Mom" in this script can be changed for any individual whose absence causes the child anxiety. Parents, teachers, and caregivers should prompt children to use this exercise anytime they feel separation anxiety. After the exercise has been practiced sufficiently, adults may cue the child to simply "do your exercise" or "take a big breath and count to three." This exercise can be modified from the school environment to any other appropriate environment.

Here are some suggested therapeutic procedures.

1. Tell me three good things about your mom/caregiver. Do these ever go away? Are they still there when she is not with you?

2. Remember in the exercise when you felt relaxed and happy? What did you do to feel happy? What did you say to yourself to feel relaxed? When you did this, you did it all by yourself, right? When your mom/caregiver was not next to you, you could say it in your heart, "I feel happy because I will see my mom later. I feel happy because I am brave." Let's practice: "I feel happy even though my mom is not next to me. I feel happy because I am brave at school."

B12

Test-Anxiety Relief

Laura Tolle

This script is for fourth, fifth, and sixth graders who have high test anxiety. The imagery begins with relaxation, then goes into a story about taking a test while giving positive self-messages to get the recipients in the right frame of mind (success regardless of test performance). After the story, there is a short period of relaxation. The goal of this imagery is to guide students through the entire process of taking a test in a calm state.

Upon completion of the imagery, each individual will process his or her thoughts and feelings. To maximize effectiveness, use this imagery after several therapeutic sessions that targeted test anxiety.

Script

Find a comfortable position. Now close your eyes and try to relax. Take a deep breath. Imagine walking down a beach, in the early morning. Feel the sand between your toes and the cool water running over your feet. Listen as the water crashes over the land. As you glance out over the calm blue water, you see the sun rising and its bright orange reflection shining across the water. Now feel the warm breeze that's blowing across your face. In the distance, you see sailboats dropping anchor and getting ready to fish for the day. Back on the beach you watch the seagulls searching for food, and you carefully listen as they talk with each other. Now imagine that you stop walking. You spot a log on the beach, and you decide to run over to it and sit down. Take a deep breath and let it out slowly. Think of this wonderful place as a secure place, somewhere you can go to escape the pressures of daily life.

Now that you are relaxed, I'm going to tell you a story. Imagine that you are the person I'm telling you about. It's Friday, and you are about to head toward English class to take that famous weekly spelling test. As you approach the room, you begin to tell yourself: "I know my spelling words because I studied hard"; "I will put every effort into this test"; "I will be proud of the grade I receive"; "I won't let anyone down; they will accept me regardless of what grade I make on this test." Now you are standing at the door. Open the door and go in. Walk to your desk. Sit at your desk and talk with your neighbors like you would on any day. The teacher gets the attention of the class and says it's time to begin. Take a deep breath. You put your books away and take out your test pencil.

Now I'm going to count to five. As you listen to the numbers, take a deep breath. Ready, 1, 2, 3, 4, and 5. Good, now slowly let it out. Tell yourself, "I'm ready for this test!" Notice that you do not feel overwhelmed or nervous or have those shaky legs. Take a deep breath again. The teacher gives you the first word. You focus and listen to the word. Now the teacher waits a minute for the class to write down the word. Before writing down the word, you sound it out in your head. With ease, you grasp your pencil and write it on the paper. The teacher proceeds with the remainder of the words. You sound each word out in your head before writing it down. Once you have envisioned the word, write it on your paper. The last word has been given to you, and you gladly write it down. You put your pencil away. The teacher asks that the tests be handed forward. You hand your test in and glance around the room at your friends' expressions. Take another deep breath and say to yourself "I did it! I successfully completed this test without anxiety!"

Now the weekend is over and you are back in school. You are going to English class. You are eager to know how you did on that spelling test. Your teacher welcomes everyone back to school and states that she is going to hand your spelling test back. She approaches you and hands the graded test to you. Before you look at the test, take a deep breath. Now look at the test. You realize that you missed two out of the twenty spelling words. A big smile appears on your face. You can't wait to tell your friends and family how well you did. In addition to your good grade, the teacher gives you a sticker on the test. You are so pleased with this test that when you get home, you put it on the refrigerator. Not only are you excited about the grade, but you are also proud of the fact that you completed a test without anxiety. You are now one step closer to approaching and taking tests without anxiety. Congratulations!

We've now reached the end of our story. Take a deep breath. Slowly open your eyes. Now slowly stand up and reach your hands toward the sky and stretch. OK, now take another deep breath and relax.

Application

This exercise assists students who experience anxiety and nervousness when taking a test. After the exercise, ask the student the following questions as a means to find ways to achieve the greatest level of calmness.

1. How does it feel to approach a test in a calm manner?
2. Was there any time in the story that you felt anxious and felt that you could not go on? When?
3. What is the difference between being calm and being anxious?
4. Take a deep breath now, slowly in, 1, 2, 3, and out. How does this feel now? How does this deep breath differ from those in the exercise?
5. What would you do to prepare for your next test, so that you would not feel anxious?

The Other Side of the Rainbow

Heather Alden Pope

This exercise is for children and adolescents who have been victims of abuse, trauma, or domestic violence. It is recommended that the child sit on a colorful blanket during the exercise. After the session, give the child a piece of cloth to keep as a tactile reminder of the journey to another place.

In this exercise, the imagery of a safe place to play reminds clients that they are children. The script involves making choices as a means of empowering the children to actively participate in their journey. The tactile component is intended to remind clients of their ability to use their minds and "travel" outside of their reality. The story includes some potentially stressful encounters that turn out to be wonderful surprises along the way. This script is best used after a relationship has been established, as the story's success depends on the level of trust between the child and the therapist. Stop the exercise at any time if the child shows significant signs of distress. Process any upsetting feelings before continuing.

Script

Find a comfortable place to sit where you are not crowded and feel relaxed. In the middle of this exercise, I will ask you to say something. When you hear "Just tell me what your choice is," give me your answer at that time. It's OK not to give an answer, or to give your answer within your heart. Remember, we can stop at any time if you choose to. If you are ready to begin, close your eyes.

Close your eyes gently and take a deep breath. Allow all your thoughts and worries to escape one by one out of your mind. Take another deep breath, and see your favorite color in the rainbow. Now fill your mind with your favorite color. Visualize yourself standing at the end of this rainbow and looking up into the sky. This rainbow is going to be the staircase that you and I will climb. We will travel to the other side of the rainbow, to the land beyond the stars. Together we are going to visit a very special place where you will be able to run, jump, play, and be safe. Are you ready?

OK, now let's get ready to climb. To climb the rainbow, first wrap your arms around your favorite color—it may be red, orange, yellow, green, blue, indigo, or violet. Hold on tightly, and think of good things about yourself. This will give us the energy we need to climb the rainbow. When you are ready, nod your head. OK, here we go, hold on tightly, start thinking good thoughts, think harder . . . You are a special child. You are smart. You are talented. You have a bright future ahead of you. Can you feel yourself lifting into the air? You can be anything that you want to be. You can dream. You are cared for. You are valuable. I can see you rounding the arch toward the top . . . Hold on tightly! You are loved. We are going to start sliding down into a wonderfully magical place. Hold on until we have landed safely. OK, here we are, you can let go. THUMP.

Feel the lush grass beneath your feet. This grass is a beautiful shade of green and feels very squishy under your toes. Are you ready to go exploring? First of all, let's follow along the purple path; it will take us to a fabulous playground where all children are safe to play. There is no one around here who wants to hurt you—you are protected here. This is a special place where you are free to laugh, jump, run, and swing! Let's continue.

In front of you, there is a huge playground filled with brightly colored equipment—slides, jungle gyms, merry-go-rounds, swings, a rope bridge, a teeter-totter, and lots of mats to jump on. Everywhere you look, children are playing. The air is filled with the sounds of their laughter. The sky is a brilliant blue, and the birds are singing in a nearby tree. Go ahead, run and play. I will be sitting on this bench while you enjoy yourself. You spin round and round on the merry-go-round. After you feel dizzy, you jump off and run over to the jungle gym. Arm over arm you swing on the bars. Some children are playing tag and invite you to join them. You look at me, and I smile encouragingly. You play with your new friends, and your laughter mixes with theirs, filling the air. After awhile, you run over to me and ask me to push you on the swing. "Sure, I would be happy to push you on the swing." You get on the swing and pump your legs. You go high into the sky like a bird. You smile and laugh. I can tell that you feel safe here. You are completely safe from harm. I can see that you are beginning to relax and enjoy your time on this side of the rainbow.

[Stop here to process feelings if necessary. Afterward, continue the exercise or wait to start again in the next session.]

Are you ready to keep exploring this magical place? The path divides right here; do you want to go to the gingerbread house or the ol' swimming hole? Continue to keep your eyes closed. Just tell me what your choice is [Wait until the child makes a choice. If no choice is made, use either one.] Great choice, wave good-bye to your new friends. Let's go and continue our grand adventure.

The Gingerbread House

This is the path to the magical gingerbread house. Let's follow along the stone path into the woods. Don't worry. The woods are filled with tall trees, squirrels, birds, rabbits, and foxes, all welcoming you to their home. Can't you hear them chattering? They seem to be delighted to meet you. Wow, what a beautiful day! You skip along the path, and after you turn the bend, there is the most inviting home you have ever seen. It looks good enough to eat. Are you hungry? I always have room for chocolate! Let's visit the owner of this beautiful house; I know that she would love to meet you! You knock on the front door, and a woman with silvery gray hair and pink, rosy cheeks answers the door. She leans down to look you in the eye and welcome you to her home. "Welcome, [child's name], it is so nice to meet you! [Your name], it is great to see you again as well! What brings you to my side of the rainbow?" "Well, [child's name] and I are on an adventure to the land beyond the stars. Today we are concentrating on having fun and celebrating that there is not one person who will hurt us here."

"Well," says the old woman, "you are welcome to come in. I have just finished baking a chocolate cake. Would you like some?" We follow her into her home and are welcomed by a room full of flowering plants, a large piano, and lots of fabulous toys. Beyond this room is the patio.

We walk out to the patio and see the petting zoo that fills the backyard. There are many animals: lambs, kittens, puppies, ponies, and baby ducks swimming with their mom in the pond. The air is filled with the sounds of happy animals, and you rush toward them to play. The animals all clamber over to get your attention. The old woman joins us and gives you some food to feed the animals. The lamb sits on your lap while the puppies roll around next to you. The old woman motions to the pony and introduces you to Applejack. The old woman invites you to ride Applejack around in the yard. You look at me and I smile, "You are welcome to ride if you want to!" You eagerly nod your head and climb onto Applejack's back. The old woman leads you around the yard, and the air is filled with the sound of your laughter. What a magnificent day! After some time, I motion for you to return because it is time to leave. You get off Applejack and feed her some hay while we slice the cake.

We join the old woman for a piece of delicious chocolate cake. After saying our good-byes, we head back along the path through the forest to the playground.

As you skip along the path toward the playground, the birds' songs fill the air. The sun is beginning to slide toward the horizon, and it is getting time to head back. We reach the rainbow, and its colorful beauty rises before us. I remind you of our special journey to this side of the rainbow. We talk about all of the beauty we have seen and the fun we have had.

As we reach for the rainbow, you hugging your favorite color and I mine, we gently slide back down toward our real lives. As we near the bottom, I look at you and smile. I have enjoyed watching you play, laugh, jump, and run around. I hope that you can always remember that mental journeys are often possible. We reach the bottom of the rainbow and turn toward this room. Now we are back in this room, and the rainbow has faded away.

When you open your eyes, I will give you a piece of cloth to remind you of the rainbow and the land beyond the stars. This cloth can take you far away if you only close your eyes and believe. Remember that there are safe places where you are loved and cared for, places where you can be a child and be safe. While you may not see them with your open eyes, if you close your eyes, your mind can take you there.

The Ol' Swimming Hole

There's the long, winding path to the ol' swimming hole. As we head down the path toward the river, we can hear lots of giggles and squeals followed by large splashes. You are getting excited, and you look to me to see if you can run ahead. I smile and nod as you pick up your pace with excitement. The day is warming up, and a cool splash in the water will feel very refreshing. Luckily there are swimsuits and towels available at the lifeguard stand next to the swimming area. When I arrive, you have already been there a few minutes, and you have started to explore the area. The swimming hole is very large and has several large oak trees with tire swings dangling over the water. We watch the kids swing from the tires into the water. It looks like great fun! There are changing rooms available, so I send you off to change into a swimsuit.

You decide that rather than easing into the cool water, jumping in would be more fun! You find an empty tire swing and swing back and forth a couple of times before you have the nerve to jump in. "Wow, the water is freezing!" you yelp as you explode from the surface. I laugh and smile. It is fun to see you so happy and carefree. All around you are children of your age playing in the water. They are delighted to meet you and invite you to join in their games. You look at me, and I smile and say, "I will be right here watching you." Over and over again you swing from the tree into the water. Sometimes you go alone, and sometimes your new friends swing with you on the same tire. It looks like great fun. The cool sprays of water keep me cool while I sit in the shade of the oak trees. I can see that you are not worrying about anything other than how quickly you can climb out of the water and get back on a swing. I am pleased to see that you are laughing and that nothing seems to be bothering you!

When you are tired out, you join me on the bank, where I have some snacks and soda for each of us. We relax and enjoy the chips and cookies while we sip our sodas. After you dry off and change, we need to head back toward the playground. You wave good-bye to all your newfound friends, and we walk together through the woods toward the playground.

As you skip along the path toward the playground, the birds' songs fill the air. The sun is beginning to slide toward the horizon, and it is getting time to head back. We reach the rainbow, and its colorful beauty rises before us. I remind you of our special journey to this side of the rainbow. We talk about all the beauty we have seen and the fun we have had.

As we reach for the rainbow, you hugging your favorite color and I mine, we gently slide back down toward our real lives. As we near the bottom, I look at you and smile. I have enjoyed watching you play, laugh, jump, and run around.

I hope that you can always remember that mental journeys are often possible. We reach the bottom of the rainbow and turn toward this room. Now we are back in this room, and the rainbow has faded away.

After you open your eyes, I will give you a piece of cloth to remind you of the rainbow and the land beyond the stars. This cloth can take you far away if you only close your eyes and believe. Remember that there are safe places where you are loved and cared for. Places where you can be a child and be safe. While you may not see them with your open eyes, if you close your eyes, your mind can take you there.

Application

In order to create a safe environment for the child, accompany the child in the scenes. If there is a trusted adult in the child's life, replace "I" with this individual in the script. In processing this imagery session, the child could draw a picture of what he or she "saw" on the other side of the rainbow, discuss what it was like to walk through the woods and meet all the new children at the playground or the swimming hole. The child can also talk about what he or she saw and what he or she was proud of (e.g., playing freely, meeting new people, riding a pony for the first time, walking through the woods, climbing the actual rainbow).

Guided Imagery for
Families and Groups

Anger Control and Relaxation

Michele Ostrowski Taylor

The exercise is for groups of children aged four to eleven who experience out-of-control or excessive anger. It can show children ways to relax and control anger at a time when they are not actively angry by giving them control over an imaginary anger creature. It is important to stress to children that they are safe in this exercise. This exercise can be used once or repeatedly, depending on the child's response and the exercise's effectiveness.

Script

Lie down or sit so that you are comfortable. Now take a deep breath and watch your stomach move up and down. Good. Now take three more slow, deep breaths and watch your stomach move up and down. 1 . . . 2 . . . 3 . . . Good. Now close your eyes and take five more deep breaths while feeling your stomach move up and down. 1 . . . breathe in, and out . . . 2 . . . in, and out . . . 3 . . . feel your stomach move up, and down . . . 4 . . . breathe in slowly, and out . . . and 5 . . . in, and out. That feels good.

Picture yourself going to a special place—a safe place. You feel calm and safe. Now we are going to make up an imaginary creature—a make-believe creature called the Anger Thing. Picture this creature in your mind—it looks like you feel when you are very, very angry. Make a really tight fist and picture the Anger Thing across the room or far away from you. It is enormous, but you are in your safe place, just watching it from far away. [Pause.] Now feel your tight fist relax, and shake your hands and fingers in the air.

The Anger Thing seems to be shrinking very slowly. Take a deep breath—breathe in slowly . . . and let your breath out slowly . . . Good. Relax your hands again by gently shaking your fingers. As you are relaxing, the Anger Thing is getting smaller and smaller as you watch it. It is now the same size as you.

Take another deep breath while you shake your fingers and relax your hands. Now, breathe out slowly. As you watch the Anger Thing, tell it to calm down and go away. [Pause.] It is getting even smaller as you are talking to it. Tell it that you are in control and want it to stop being such an angry Thing. It is shrinking even more . . . Wiggle your fingers and toes. Now take another deep breath . . . and let it out. You look back at the Anger Thing and see that it is turning into a very small, soft and fuzzy creature—like a bunny rabbit. Tell it that it doesn't need to be so angry anymore. It comes toward you and is very friendly. You can touch it now, and feel how soft it is. That's nice. [Pause.]

Now we are going to take five deep breaths slowly, as we come back to the room. 1 . . . breathe in, and out . . . 2 . . . in, and out . . . 3 . . . feel your stomach move up, and down . . . 4 . . . breathe in slowly, and out . . . and 5 . . . in, and out. Open your eyes when you are ready.

Application

Do this exercise in a controlled setting. Depending on each child's age and response to the script, this exercise can be repeated in future sessions or at home by the child and the child's caretaker. Discuss the experience with each child to find out his or her reaction to the exercise, and use the exercise as a teaching tool to help each child calm down when angry.

Always talk to the parents or guardians before trying this exercise, so that they will be aware of what will take place. Also, assess the childrens' susceptibility to nightmares before trying this exercise. If a child has nightmares after doing this exercise, discontinue its use immediately. Parents or guardians can help monitor the effects and reinforce positive learning from it. Questions to explore include the following:

1. What did your Anger Thing look like?
2. How did it feel when you could control the Anger Thing and make it smaller?
3. Could you do the same thing when you feel angry?
4. What are some things you could do to control your angry feelings?
5. What would you suggest to children of your age to do to control anger?

B15

Building Self-Esteem

Amy L. Thompson

This guided imagery is for a group of children or adolescents who need help improving their self-esteem. It combines self-affirmations with visualization. It is a general-purpose exercise to help clients feel more confident and change the way they view themselves. Alter the script to include any scenario that will help clients improve their self-image or change the way they relate to others. It can also be used to accomplish a very specific goal by visualizing a scene using positive action and to achieve a positive outcome.

This exercise can be done with any age group, as long as the scenarios are age-appropriate. It is also conducive to clients of various cultural backgrounds, given an assessment of cultural expectations.

Script

Sit in a comfortable chair, or lie on the bed or on the floor. Relax. [Pause three seconds.] Close your eyes. [Pause three seconds.] Let go of all your thoughts. Breathe in, hold it [pause three seconds], and let it out. Good. Again, one more. That's right. Feel yourself relax. Feel the stress leave your body.

Imagine this scene: You're taking a day off from work or school. You feel comfortable about yourself. You're getting dressed in your favorite clothes. See the colors of the clothes. Feel the textures as you slowly put on each article of clothing. Tell yourself, "I deserve nice things, and I deserve to feel good."

Go to the mirror. Admire your clothes. See how nice you look in them. Stand up straight and feel how clean and refreshed your skin feels under the clothes, how strong your muscles feel when you stand straight. Tell yourself, "I look fine."

Fix your hair the way you like it. Adjust your collar. Smile at yourself in the mirror. Actually feel the muscles in your face form the smile. Look at yourself smiling and notice how much more open and relaxed you look when you smile. When you see the parts of your appearance you usually don't like, notice that they seem less dominant, less important. If a self-critical thought comes to mind, let it pass. Tell yourself, "I am OK just as I am."

Now go into the kitchen. See the kitchen in detail: the stove, the cabinets, and the sink. Go to the refrigerator and open it. See it full of nutritious, appealing food. Look in the cabinets and see good food you would like to prepare for yourself. Tell yourself, "I've got what I need."

Prepare a simple dish for yourself, something delicious and good for you. It could be a salad, some soup, or a nutritious sandwich. Take your time and enjoy the process of getting out the ingredients, slicing bread or vegetables, warming up the soup, and arranging things attractively on the plate. Tell yourself, "I deserve to eat well."

See the colors, feel the temperatures and textures, smell the enticing aromas. Admire the dish you have made for yourself. Tell yourself, "I am good at doing things for myself."

Eat your food, sitting down quietly at the table and taking your time. Linger over each bite, really tasting each bite. When you are finished, feel how full and comfortable you feel, how you are nourished and at peace with life. Let a feeling of contentment come over you. Tell yourself, "I love myself. I take care of myself."

Clean up after yourself. As you are cleaning, drop a cup or a plate and break it. Say, "Oh well, it's no big deal." If derogatory labels pop into your mind like "stupid" or "clumsy" or "bad," cut them off. Tell yourself, "I allow myself to make mistakes. I'm OK just as I am."

Now get ready to leave your home. You are going for a leisurely walk. Go outside and walk down the street. It is a sunny day, warm and pleasant. Enjoy the feel of your muscles moving, your lungs breathing the fresh, pure air, the warmth of the sun on your shoulders. Notice how bright, crisp, and clear everything looks. Hear the sound of birds, a dog barking in the distance, cars going by, music playing on a radio somewhere. Tell yourself, "I can enjoy the simple things in life."

See someone walking toward you, a stranger or a neighbor you recognize but don't actually know. See the stranger catch your eye and smile at you. Maintain eye contact and give a small smile in return. Tell yourself, "I am willing to take risks."

Keep walking. You see another stranger approach and smile at you. This time, maintain eye contact, smile widely, and say loudly and clearly, "Hi, how are you?" Continue walking down the sidewalk, and keep smiling. Tell yourself, "I am outgoing and confident."

Now as you walk down the sidewalk, you notice a flower shop. You decide to go in and buy yourself some flowers. Look around and see all the different colors of flowers. Notice the aroma, how lovely it smells. Walk around and select several kinds of flowers to make a bouquet that you like. With the flowers in your arms, approach the salesperson and pay for them. As you leave the shop, tell yourself, "I deserve nice things. I am a valuable and worthy person."

Walk back toward your home. Appreciate the sights and sounds of the outdoors as you walk. When you get home, notice that your home is uniquely yours. Look around at all of your comforts. Tell yourself, "I am proud of what I have."

Now it is time to end our exercise. Slowly bring yourself back into this room by picturing your surroundings. Take a deep breath and count to five slowly. Slowly open your eyes. We are now finished with the exercise for today. How do you feel? Tell yourself, "I feel good about myself."

Application

After the exercise, ask how the clients felt and what they saw during the visualization. You could make a copy of the positive affirmations listed below for the clients, to use as personal daily affirmations.

1. I deserve nice things, and I deserve to feel good.
2. I look fine.
3. I am OK just as I am.
4. I've got what I need.
5. I deserve to eat well.
6. I am good at doing things for myself.
7. I love myself. I take care of myself.
8. I allow myself to make mistakes. I'm OK just as I am.
9. I can enjoy the simple things in life.
10. I am willing to take risks.
11. I am outgoing and confident.
12. I deserve nice things. I am a valuable and worthy person.
13. I am proud of what I have.
14. I feel good about myself.

Come with Me into the Field

Lori Swan Provence

This relaxation exercise can be used with almost anyone who is experiencing stress, especially those who receive little praise or positive reinforcement. Guided imagery is a wonderful therapeutic tool in that it allows clients to take a break from the stressors of daily life without ever leaving their seats. This exercise has no age, racial, cultural, or socioeconomic implications. It can be used with individuals or groups.

Script

Get into a comfortable position. Close your eyes and try to relax. Listen to the sound of your breathing. Breathe in—breathe out. Take a deep breath and let it out slowly. You are now beginning to feel more relaxed.

Picture yourself walking through a vast field. The sun is bright and high in the sky. Feel its warmth on your skin. Feel the cool green grass between your toes. Notice the wildflowers growing all around you. You are fascinated by the beautiful colors—blue, purple, gold, white—the colors are vibrant and bright.

Feel the gentle breeze as it blows through your hair. Breathe deeply and smell the wildflowers as the breeze gently wafts their scent. As you continue walking, you hear the beautiful songs of the birds that fly overhead. You find yourself chirping back to them and feeling a new appreciation for their beauty. You hear a pleasant sound in the distance, and you begin to walk toward it.

Continue breathing slowly, taking in the sights and sounds around you—good.

Notice the beauty and grace of the butterflies that flutter past you as you walk. The colors and patterns of their wings mesmerize you. The sound that brought you to this part of the field continues to draw you to it. Your pace quickens ever so slightly as the sound grows closer and closer. Suddenly you discover that the sound you were searching for is a small stream. Watch and listen as the water trickles by.

Continue breathing in—and out—excellent.

You notice schools of small fish swimming so gracefully with the flow of the water. You see a turtle sprawling from its shell to enjoy the warmth of the sun. You kneel down and dip your hands into the stream, being careful not to disturb its inhabitants. Now you cup your hands and bring some of the water to your mouth. As the cool water trickles down your throat, you feel very refreshed. You sit near the water's edge and continue to enjoy the beauty of nature that surrounds you.

Continue to breathe in—and out—very good.

You notice that the turtle has retreated into its shell and that the birds have grown quiet. The sun is still shining, but not quite as brightly as before. You realize that you have lost track of time and that you must return home now. You stand up and stretch, still breathing in—and out—taking one last look around at the beauty of what is before you.

I will now count backward from five to one to bring you back into the room: 5, continue to breathe deeply—good—4, you feel more alert and energized. 3, continue breathing in—and out—very good. 2, begin to move your fingers, toes, and shoulders. 1, open your eyes and stretch—you feel very relaxed and refreshed.

You are now back in the room with me—I hope you enjoyed your getaway.

Application

It is important to be aware of any negative experiences clients may have previously had with any of the things mentioned in this exercise (i.e., water, birds, allergies, etc.). Any negative connotations may keep this exercise from being relaxing. After the exercise, ask clients for feedback on the exercise. You can also encourage your clients to create and take a minivacation of their own when they feel particularly stressed.

Therapeutic questions can include

1. In this exercise, several positive words were used. What does the word "good" represent? How about "very good"? "Excellent"?

2. When you hear people praising you, how do you feel? What kind of praises have you received in the past? What did you do to earn these praises?

3. What do you do to relax? What symbol would you use to represent relaxation? [Probe: a fish swimming freely]

4. What would you do to bring this relaxed feeling to your school/work/home?

B17

Coping with Powerlessness

Kristin Geiss-Curran

This guided imagery is for individuals or groups of older children and adolescents. Children face a variety of difficult situations that are beyond their power to control (divorce, substance abuse, violence, loss, etc.). This exercise is helpful in exploring and discussing feelings of helplessness and frustration. It seeks to validate the inner strength and goodness of participants while helping them gain a new perspective on their situation. This exercise may relate to a wide range of issues.

Script

Get very comfortable. Let your eyes close softly. Let your body sink into your chair. Starting at the top of your head, let all of your muscles relax. Let your forehead relax, let your cheeks relax, let your jaw and neck relax. Let the relaxation melt farther down your body—your shoulders, your arms, and your fingers. All of your body is relaxing down to your waist; then allow your legs, your knees, and your feet to release. All the tension in your body has slid down into your feet, and it leaves your body through your toes. Any stress, pressure, or nervousness rushes down to the tips of your toes and flees your body. You feel empty, limp, and completely relaxed.

Any thoughts that come into your mind sink to your feet, float out of your toes, and then quickly blow up and away into the air around you. You feel limp like an empty balloon. Now breathe slowly and deeply. In through your nose, slowly the fresh air comes in, pauses for a second, and then slowly blows out of your mouth. In through your nose with the fresh, energizing air, and out with the old air. As you breathe out of your mouth, anything that enters your mind rushes out of your body with your breath; you are filled with only pure, empty space. Breathe in the healthy, pure air, and blow out any thoughts or anxieties. The clean, fresh air is so light and carefree that you begin to feel weightless. All thoughts, cares, and worries are out of your body, and the fresh air is filling you up like a balloon. As you fill up with more and more weightless, fresh air, you become lighter than all the space around you.

Your body is lifting up off the ground because it is so lightweight. You are completely at ease as you float higher and higher. Continue to breathe in the fresh, pure air, and to blow out anything heavy, tense, or distracting.

In your mind, you are a big, round balloon, filled with light air that allows you to soar through the sky up above everything else. This balloon is your favorite color. Picture yourself now. You float high above the trees and into the fluffy white clouds. You feel gentle breezes bouncing you on cushions of air. Like a feather, you move effortlessly across the sky, guided by the breeze. You cannot control the direction that the wind takes you; you simply relax and trust that the light, fresh air inside you will keep you afloat. Any worry or tension that enters your mind or body, simply blow out your mouth, and then take a deep breath of air in through your nose. Keep breathing deeply as you fly high above the ground and look around at the beautiful, blue sky, the soft, fluffy clouds, and the green earth far below.

Suddenly, a big gust of wind carries your balloon down into a tree. You are helpless to steer yourself in a different direction, but you continue to take deep breaths of fresh air, which fill you with peace. Your balloon becomes wedged in the tree's branches, no longer able to float freely through the sky. The branches of the tree are twisted and sharp, but your balloon is strong and cannot be punctured by the branches. Your balloon shell is made of a strong rubber that can stretch and bend, but it can never be broken. Imagine how it feels to have the tree branches poking into the smooth skin of your balloon.

Imagine how it feels to be suspended in that tree. Inside your balloon all the fresh, pure air is still safe and protected from harm. Continue to breathe in and out and imagine you are this balloon.

Someone is now walking to the tree, and gently trying to nudge you free. Imagine how it feels to be tugged, pulled, and pushed. You continue to breathe deeply, in with the fresh, pure air, and out with all your worries and concerns. Because your balloon is made of superstrong rubber that cannot break, you bend and change your shape as you are being pulled. As your shape changes, you are able to fit between the branches that have kept you wedged in one place. Finally, you are released from between the twisted branches. In an instant, you are free of the tree, back to your smooth round shape, and bobbing in the air. Be aware of the different feelings you have now. Look down upon the person who gave you the nudge, and notice his or her face. Breathe in more of the pure, light air and feel yourself rise into the sky. Gentle breezes are again blowing your balloon toward the clouds. You are free. You enjoy the weightless feeling as you fly up above everything and everyone.

Now a new gust of wind is blowing back to this room, back to your chair. You are floating down, down, down, and as I count backward from ten, you will sit in your chair and slowly change from the balloon to your regular self. 10, 9, 8, 7, 6 . . . open your eyes . . . 5, 4, 3, 2, 1.

Application

After the exercise, make sure the children come back to reality and don't hide their emotions in the imagery world. Invite them to speak by asking, "How do you feel?" or empower them to feel their inner strength by saying, "I'm powerful" loudly together. Then process feelings that are associated with the exercise by relating to a past experience.

1. List the thoughts and feelings that you "breathed out" during the exercise. Were there any that kept coming back again and again?

2. Does the superstrong rubber of the balloon keep out everything? What sorts of things do you want to do through the power of the balloon?

3. Describe a situation similar to this experience. What "branches" trapped you for a while? Did anyone help you free? Describe the face and feelings you experienced.

B18

Good-bye Balloon

Monit Cheung

Grieving is a painful process. It can take months and years to recover from loss, in part because feelings of grief are difficult to express. Therefore, it is important to have a formal ritual for clients to express wishes and say good-bye to their loved ones. This therapeutic exercise gives clients of all ages an opportunity to express their wishes.

First, draw four circles on a piece of paper to represent balloons and ask clients to color each of the balloons. Use a variety of colors to represent life and hope. Second, encourage them to write down wishes, unfinished businesses, and any word or statement they wish to make for the deceased or separated. Finally, use the following guided imagery as a formal ritual of saying good-bye.

Script

Sit or lie down in a comfortable position. Relax and enjoy this journey to give your loved ones a few of your wishes. These wishes are important to them.

Visualize the balloons you just saw. Remember the colors you filled in for the balloons—blue, green, yellow, red, pink, purple, black, white, orange, and other colors. Each of these colors is flying toward the sky, up, up and above, to reach someone you love and treasure. You like to see these colors moving upward. You like to see them go to your loved ones, telling them how much you love them, telling them how much you miss them.

Remember the words you put next to each balloon. They are your wishes and something you want to tell your loved ones. Imagine the entire alphabet is flying up toward the sky. A-B-C-D, E-F-G, you are flying higher and higher; H-I-J-K, L-M-N, you are flying with the balloon to the sky; O-P-Q, R-S-T, your loved one says, "I love you"; U-V-W, X-Y-Z, now you want to read your wishes louder and louder from your heart.

Visualize the first wish. [Read it aloud.] Repeat this wish in your heart. [Pause.] Here we go! This wish goes up with the balloon to the sky, reaching your loved ones in a wonderful place. They enjoy reading it. It is a good wish! Relax and enjoy!

Here is your second wish. [Read it aloud.] Repeat this wish in your heart. [Pause.] This wish is flying with a colorful balloon. It is going to reach your loved ones in a beautiful place. It is a wish from your heart. Relax!

Your third wish is [read it aloud.] Repeat this wish in your heart. [Pause.] Now you can release it with a beautiful balloon to the sky. Imagine the sky is blue and the balloon is brightly colored. Your wish goes up and up. It is wonderful!

Now you are saying good-bye. Good-bye, good-bye, good-bye . . . All the balloons are now gone. They are reaching your loved ones. They are going to release all your wishes, your sadness, your good-byes.

Remember all the colors on the balloons—blue, green, yellow, red, pink, purple, black, white, orange, and other colors. Remember all the letters on your balloons—A, B, C, D, E, F, G, H, I, J, K, L, M, N, O, P, Q, R, S, T, U, V, W, X, Y, and Z—slowly one by one going to the sky, reaching your loved ones. You are relaxed and feel happy now. Your mind is clear, and your heart is full of love.

When the numbers go from ten to one, you are ready to open your eyes and feel refreshed. 10, 9, 8, 7, 6, open your eyes. 5, 4, 3, 2, 1, you are back to this room and you are feeling great!

Application

This exercise can be used in any grieving situation. The script can be modified to suit the needs of the client. Coloring the balloons before this exercise is necessary to facilitate the visual imagery of the balloons. In a family session, encourage all family members to contribute to the coloring and writing process. After the guided imagery is over, the family can keep the balloon sheet to remember the experience. Alternatively, they can tear the sheet into small pieces to symbolize ending the grieving process.

B19

Let the Tension Go
Yolanda Alvarado

This exercise can be used for groups or individuals of any age. It helps clients who have trouble concentrating to focus on the therapeutic effect during a counseling session. It also offers a way to relax and feel more peaceful after describing a painful memory. If possible, use soft music in the background. Ask clients to clear their minds of all unnecessary and stressful thoughts and to find a comfortable position.

Script

First, find a focal point. This can be any item or spot in the room, but it should be as far away from you as possible. After about fifteen seconds, slowly close your eyes. Or, if you wish, you may keep your eyes open, but continue to focus on your focal point. As you relax, the focal point may begin to fade, and your eyes may close naturally. [Dim the lights after clients find a concentration point in the room.]

For the next few minutes, allow yourself to relax. You've chosen to take the time to reduce the accumulated stress and tension in your body. For now, focus on the fact that you are free at this moment and that you don't have to solve any problems right now.

As this occurs, you'll notice yourself beginning to relax. Listen to the sounds reaching your ears. Be aware of the soothing music and my voice. Let the sounds give you permission to relax, to let go and relax. Become aware of your feet. Let your feet begin to relax. Let the tension drain out from your feet, drain out through the tips of your toes. As you breathe, breathe relaxation into your toes.

Let your calves relax, feel all the tension leave your calves. Feel all the tension flow out through your ankles, through your feet, and out through the tips of your toes. As you breathe, breathe relaxation into your calves.

Now let your thighs relax. Feel them become more relaxed as the tension flows out through your legs and out through the tips of your toes. Breathe relaxation throughout your legs; feel them relaxing more and more. Become aware of how each breath releases tension, releasing tension throughout your abdomen and your pelvic area. Relax, let the tension flow out through your legs, down to your feet, and out your toes.

Feel your arms relax, feel the tension draining out, draining out through your hands and out through your fingertips. Breathe relaxation into your arms, your hands, and your fingers.

Now focus on your back, shoulders, and neck. Breathe out all the tension and breathe in relaxation. Feel the tension leave your body. Relax as the tension flows out with each breath. You can also feel the muscles around your face start to relax. Feel the muscles around your mouth relax, and all the other facial muscles relax. Feel the tension lift from your face as you breathe in and breathe out relaxation.

Feel your forehead and scalp relaxing. All the tension from your head, neck, and shoulders is flowing down through your arms and hands—draining out through the tips of your fingers. Continue breathing out all the tension in your body, and breathe in relaxation. With each breath you are falling into a deeper and deeper relaxed state. If unnecessary thoughts begin to enter your mind, release them as you exhale and breathe in relaxation. As you inhale relaxation, you'll feel fresh clean air washing away all unnecessary thoughts. Allow each breath to cleanse your mind, rejuvenate it, and energize it. As you continue breathing in relaxation, imagine yourself in a familiar, safe, and tranquil place. Notice how relaxed you are in this tranquil place, and time will begin to slow down.

Time slows down, and the next few minutes seem to last a long time, and during this time, you'll feel more and more relaxed. Enjoy this time as it slowly passes. Again, become aware of how each breath brings you relaxation. Notice how you feel more rested. As each breath rejuvenates your body, notice how you're beginning to feel more energized. Become more energized and alert. Become more alert to the outside world as we begin to count to ten. 1, you're becoming more alert. 2, open your eyes and feel energized. 3, feel more and more alert. 4, prepare your body to stretch. 5, stretch your arms. 6, stretch your legs. 7, feeling even more alert. 8, feeling completely awake. 9, feeling alert and rested. 10, feel the new energy throughout your body and mind.

Now you are alert and ready to return to the outside world.

Application

Practice this exercise with clients at the beginning of a session or when clients show signs of distress. You could record the script on a tape with background music and use it as a homework assignment for clients who are self-directed. Because this exercise aims to help clients concentrate, it is important that they process the concentration point after the exercise and discuss how the problem has shifted their focus and distracted their attention.

Magic Carpet Ride
Molly Grimmer

This imagery is for groups of children who are having difficulties with their parents, but it can be used for other purposes as well, such as anxiety and separation anxiety. The exercise has two parts. The first is a relaxation exercise that will help the child learn to relax through deep breathing and tension release. The second part is a guided imagery exercise involving a magic carpet ride to a special place. This will help children discover a self-soothing place inside themselves that will help them feel less anxious.

Note: Modify this exercise for children with height phobias by shortening the carpet ride time, then increasing it gradually each time you use the exercise.

Script

Take off your shoes, and sit or lie down in a comfortable position. You may close your eyes or leave them open. Do whichever is more comfortable for you. Take a deep breath. Breathe in through your nose and out through your mouth. Again, breathe in . . . hold it . . . 1, 2, 3, 4 . . . and out. Very good. Stretch out your fingers, now relax them. Stretch them out, now relax. Feel all the tension in your body flow out through your fingertips. Breathe in . . . and out. Breathe deeply again, and when you breathe out, push out any tension that might be left in your body. Breathe in . . . and breathe out. Very good. You feel very relaxed and calm. You feel safe and secure. Continue breathing in and out. Very comfortable. Very relaxed.

Imagine that there is a magic carpet in front of you. This magic carpet can fly, and it will take you anywhere you want to go. Look at the beautiful colors in the carpet. Sit or lie down on the carpet. Feel how soft and comfortable the carpet feels beneath you. You feel the carpet slowly rise off the ground. It moves higher off the ground. You can look down off the carpet and see the ground. You feel safe and secure because you cannot fall off the carpet. This magic carpet begins to slowly move forward . . . It is moving a little faster now . . . You feel the wind blow softly across your face and through your hair. You feel calm and relaxed and safe.

The magic carpet is taking you to your special place now. This is a place that only you know about. It is a place where you feel calm and happy. You are safe and relaxed in your special place. You can see your special place in the distance. The magic carpet is coming nearer . . . and nearer . . . to your special place.

You are now in your special place. You feel the magic carpet slowly lower to the ground. You can walk around in your special place and explore . . . You can smell your special place . . . it smells so good here! You can touch things in your special place . . . feel your special place. Look at everything in your place . . . you are in your special place . . . Enjoy your place . . . [Pause for ten seconds.]

It is time to leave your special place. Look around and remember this place. Remember how it looks . . . how it smells . . . how it feels . . . remember how you feel . . . You see the magic carpet again. You go to the carpet and sit or lie down on it. Feel the carpet against your body. It's so soft! You feel the carpet slowly rise up. You can look at the ground as it rises higher and higher into the air. You are relaxed, and you know that you are safe. The carpet slowly moves forward. You feel the wind in your hair and on your face as the magic carpet brings you back. You can see the room in the distance. It is getting closer and closer. You feel the magic carpet slowly lower to the ground. Take a deep breath . . . 9 . . . 8 . . . 7 . . . take another deep breath . . . 6 . . . stretch your body . . . 5 . . . 4 . . . open your eyes . . . 3 . . . deep breath . . . 2 . . . and 1. Your eyes are open and you feel very relaxed and calm. You did very well. Now you are back and relaxed!

Application

Use this exercise when rapport and trust have been established in a therapeutic relationship. Children must feel comfortable, as the purpose of this exercise is to help them learn to relax themselves when they feel anxious. After completing the exercise, children should draw pictures or write statements about this special place. They can keep this to help them focus on their inner calm when they feel anxious. Remember that children's special places should be kept private, so do not directly ask them to share the specifics of their place unless they volunteer the information. Instead, ask,

1. How did you feel when you reached your special place?
2. What makes this place special?
3. How is this special feeling different from any other feelings?
4. Would your parents understand the soothing effect of this special place? How would you tell them if I want them to know?

Mental and Physical Relaxation

Othea G. McCoy-Clinton

Use this exercise for mature adolescents or parents who are working through parent-child relationship issues. It can be used with individuals or groups. The imagery helps clients relax and refocus through the use of music and pleasant thoughts. Select an instrumental piece of music that contains smooth and soothing combinations of sounds. Instruct clients not to tense any muscle to the point of pain or discomfort.

Script

Position yourself in a comfortable sitting or lying position. You may remove shoes for comfort and freedom. Start the music. Close your eyes tightly and take a deep breath and hold it . . . 1, 2, 3. Exhale slowly and release the tension in your eyelids. Clench your teeth and inhale. [Pause.] Now slowly exhale and relax your jaw muscles. Make a fist and inhale deeply. [Pause.] Exhale and release your fist. Move your fingers slowly and then allow your hands to relax. Inhale deeply, hold it. [Pause.] Exhale slowly through your mouth. Allow yourself to hear the calming sounds of music. Now picture yourself in a peaceful place where only music can be heard. [Pause.] It can be on the beach, in a field surrounded by wildflowers, driving down a long scenic highway with mountains in the distance. Inhale, smell the air, fragrant and sweet, green and fresh, and exhale. [Repeat several times.] Allow your body to feel the music as you allow yourself to be taken away. Your mind and body are taken by the beautiful music to that special place.

Now listen as I tell the story of change as it evolves with six great men. One day while walking through a park under a tall oak tree, Einstein was pondering the theory of relativity. Thinking aloud he said to himself, "Does it matter how a person thinks?" Unbeknown to him, Gandhi sat looking at the blue sky and responded, "Why, of course; how one thinks affects one's beliefs." Then Socrates, who sat staring at the leaves, said, "Yes, and man's beliefs influence his expectations." Exploring the tree branches was Plato, who stated that "One's expectations temper one's attitude." Then, as if on cue, Aristotle spoke, stating that "one's attitude determines one's behavior." "Ah yes, my friend," Thurgood Marshall said, "One's behavior affects one's performance." Then Einstein spoke: "Well, with all of your kind advice, we can now conclude that one's performance affects one's life, and that with all things being relative, it must be true that what one thinks rests entirely on *you*." [Music continues.]

Application

The combination of relaxation and imagery exercise is a good way to help adolescents understand the importance of maintaining a calm feeling during discussion of an important topic. The story of change can stimulate discussions about parent-child communication focusing on values and judgments. The following questions are suggested:

1. What do you think about this story?
2. Do you know the people in this story? What do they represent?
3. When a child does not agree with his or her parent, what would the parent think or feel?
4. If you were a parent, how would you punish a child when she or he was doing something wrong?
5. What is change? Do parents change if they have to? If your parents have to change something, what change is easy to make and what change is hard to make?

B22

Muscle-Group Relaxation

Monit Cheung

This exercise is designed for groups of children, adolescents, or families and can be used for relaxation in fifteen-minute periods twice a day, especially after a long day of work or school. Its purpose is to help clients compare two extreme feelings of tension and relaxation, so that they can learn how to control their temper. Clients first concentrate on the feeling of muscle tension, and contrast it with the sensation of relaxation. Instruct clients not to tense any muscle to the point of pain or discomfort. Tell clients to be especially careful with any muscle that has ever been injured. It may be necessary to consult a physician regarding the suitability of this exercise to the client's current health situation. If the client is pregnant, do not follow this procedure; just instruct the client to close her eyes and relax.

Script

Sit in a comfortable position. Take off your shoes. [Pause five seconds.] Close your eyes gently. When you do the following exercise, you will hold each of the sixteen muscle groups in tension for five to seven seconds. You will concentrate on how the tension feels in your muscles. Then, after relaxing your muscles, you will concentrate on the sensation of relaxation. Be sure to relax completely before going on to the next muscle group. Let's begin now.

1, Hands: Move the right-hand fingers quickly [pause three seconds], relax. Move your left-hand fingers quickly [pause three seconds], relax. Now make a right fist, relax. Make a left fist, relax and feel the difference. Good.

2, Upper arms: Bend your elbows and place your fingers on your shoulders. Tense your biceps for five seconds, 1, 2, 3, 4, 5. Release the tension and feel how relaxed you are now. Very good.

3, Lower arms: Hold both arms out, stretch, and then relax. Put them back next to you. Notice that they feel really good.

4, Forehead: Open your eyes. Wrinkle your forehead up. Now close your eyes and relax your forehead.

5, Eyes: Close your eyes tightly. Now open them and roll your eyes clockwise, then counterclockwise. Now close your eyes gently and relax.

6, Jaw: Open your mouth as wide as you can. Open more. Good. Open and shut your mouth and notice your jaw's movement. Do it again five times. 1, 2, 3, 4, 5. Close your mouth gently and relax.

7, Tongue: Press your tongue on the roof of your mouth toward your front teeth. Hold it. Now release.

8, Mouth: Press your lips tightly together. Now release. Feel the tension around your cheeks melting away. Relax.

9, Neck: Sit up. Bend your head toward your chest. Press your chin toward your chest. Now, facing the front again, move your right ear toward your right shoulder. Then move your left ear toward your left shoulder. Relax and enjoy your quiet environment.

10, Shoulders: Now bring both your shoulders upward toward your ears. Shrug and move the shoulders around. Relax and take a deep breath.

11, Chest: Take another deep breath. 1, slowly take a deep—breath, 2, hold it and feel the tension inside, 3, exhale slowly and feel the relaxation. Good.

12, Abdomen: Now tighten your stomach and abdominal muscles until they feel hard and strong. Release and relax. Enjoy the sensation of relaxation!

13, Back: Straighten your back and tighten your back muscles. Put your hands on your waist and take a deep breath. 1, 2, 3, exhale. Put your hands to your side and relax. Well done!

14, Hips: Gently press your hips down in your chair. Release and relax.

15, Thighs: Press your heels into the floor. Release and relax.

16, Legs: Extend your legs in front of you. Point your toes away from your body. Return to your original position. Do it again, and this time, point your toes back toward your body. Feel the tension and relax. Feel how good your muscles feel now. Take another deep breath. 1, 2, 3, exhale. Good.

Now slowly open your eyes. Stand up and stretch. You have just finished the muscle-group relaxation exercise. See you next time.

Application

Work on the first exercise with clients, in a controlled setting. After this exercise, ask the clients, "How do you feel now? Do any muscle groups give you deeper relaxation than others?" Encourage clients to focus on the most effective muscle groups when they feel tense or are about to lose their temper. Clients may complete the entire exercise before going to bed.

To evaluate the effectiveness of this exercise, use this scale (fig. B22.1) each time before and after the exercise.

Fig. B22.1 Effectiveness scale

Date _____ Time _____ a.m./p.m.				
Before the exercise, I feel				
Extremely tense	Very tense	OK	Very relaxed	Extremely relaxed
1	2	3	4	5

Date _____ Time _____ a.m./p.m.				
After the exercise, I feel				
Extremely tense	Very tense	OK	Very relaxed	Extremely relaxed
1	2	3	4	5

Ocean Walk

Patricia R. Palmer

Prerecord this exercise as a relaxation and guided imagery tape for adolescents who have experienced conflict in the family. This exercise is an empowering tool to help clients relate a beautiful natural setting to peace and joy. It encourages listeners to experience their inner strength and seek inner peace. The script has a total playing time of approximately twenty minutes. Music is an integral part of the journey and can be used to accompany the script.

Script

In this exercise, you will be going through a relaxation and guided imagery experience to help you access your own capacity for strength, joy, and peace. Please find a comfortable place to sit. Position yourself so your back is supported. Let your shoulders and arms relax and your hands rest on your lap or by your sides. Place your feet on the ground with your legs uncrossed. Gently close your eyes if you wish. Now slowly take a deep breath and let it out quietly. Take another deep breath, feel your belly rise and your chest expand, and then let the air flow out. Again, take a deep breath and let it out when you feel ready. Take one more breath and be aware of your body and the soft rhythm of your movements. Continue to breathe while you let go of all your worries and duties. Your body and spirit are ready for the journey that lies ahead.

You are walking by a gentle, quickly flowing stream. [Add music here.] You hear the water rippling over the rocks and the birds singing. It is a beautiful day. You feel the sun warming your body all over. You belong here in these lovely woods. You walk along the stream with great joy, anticipating seeing the ocean that lies just ahead around the bend in the path.

The ocean stretches out on both sides as far as you can see. The sun's rays dance on the blue water. A soft wind carries the smell of the sea to you. You stand relaxed with feet firmly on the ground and feel the earth's energy through your body. The rolling waves call you to the water's edge. You take off your shoes and socks and place them safely at the base of a rock. The warm sand tickles the soles of your feet. Listen to the sea and feel the energy of the ocean waves move across the sand to caress your feet. Breathe slowly and deeply while you feel the earth's nourishment through your body. Walk slowly toward the waves with the warmth of the sun and the sand enclosing you.

Walk into the waves. Your movements are slow and graceful, and the waves come to meet you, bathing your ankles in sun-warmed water.

You turn toward some rocks in the distance. Walk along the water's edge, feeling the warmth of water, sun, and sand. You belong in this beautiful world that surrounds you. Listen to the sound of the waves. You, too, make beautiful sounds as your feet gently splash in the water. Feel the water as it playfully grabs you and then runs away. Feel the sand moving beneath your feet as the waves retreat. Breathe deeply and inhale the spirit of the ocean through your body, into your heart. You are strong and joyful like the ocean. Bend down and dip into the water with your hands. Let the seaweed dance through your fingers and flow away. Pick up a small shell and look at the delicate patterns it holds. You have all the time you need to enjoy the beauty around you. Walk along the water's edge and awaken to the wholeness and energy of the world of which you are a part. You have all you need, too. Your spirit has the energy to do what your joyful heart chooses. The energy of the sun and sea touch your spirit, and you long to run along the shore, to express the strength and the joy you have. Stand quietly on the warm sand and feel your energy dancing through your legs. Focus on the energy as it goes through your body and up to your heart, moving you to burst forth into a joyful run.

Feel the wind softly caressing your sun-warmed body as you run along the beach. Your movements are graceful, and your feet make splashing noises when the waves come in. The sand is a soft cushion for your feet. You spring forward with each step, moved by the strength and joy within you. Feel the energy of the sun and the ocean and the wind. Feel the energy within your body and spirit. You are one with the world around you.

Feel the sun's rays dancing on your body. Feel the waves of light tingling your face and arms and legs. Warmth soothes your body, and the sun's pulse beats in your heart. Feel the wind's gentle coolness, like a soft scarf wiping your brow. Feel the energy of the wind as it soothes you with an ocean mist. You have all that you need—warmth and coolness—strength and peace. You are whole and complete like the sun and the ocean and the wind. Feel the welcoming firmness of the earth on your feet as you run. Slow down now and let the earth that has nourished you offer a place to rest. Lie down on the sandy blanket the earth has prepared for you.

The earth cradles your body in the curves of the sand. Feel your body coming to stillness. Picture the earth and sun nourishing you; picture the strength within your spirit. Your heart is filled with peace and joy. Rest here quietly as long as you wish. When you are ready, walk along the water's edge back where you first came down to the waves.

Feel the energy of the ocean, the wind, and the sun. You, too, are strong. Feel the tickle of the rolling waves and the caress of the wind. You are joyful and peaceful, too. Your spirit has the energy to do what your joyful heart chooses. Walk slowly back across the warm sand toward the woods. Pick up your shoes and socks where you left them at the base of the rock. Put them on and walk back through the beautiful woods. You are ready to bring peace, strength, and joy into your daily life. You can return to the ocean for nourishment whenever you choose. Listen quietly and open your eyes when you feel ready.

Application

This exercise can be used after intense discussions related to family conflict in individual or group sessions. Be sure to assess the suitability of using oceans as a place for relaxation before prerecording this script. Clients who have hydrophobia symptoms should not participate in this exercise without appropriate guidance by a clinical practitioner. However, this exercise can be used in conjunction with systematic desensitization. For clients who have difficulty running, the practitioner can change that part of the script to walking at a more brisk pace or dancing in the waves to express energy and joy—or can suggest that clients imagine themselves walking or dancing in place of running, if they so choose.

Therapeutic questions can focus on seeking inner peace and using coping strategies when facing difficulties in interpersonal relationships.

B24
Qigong Relaxation
Monit Cheung

Qigong (pronounced *chi-kung*) is an ancient Chinese relaxation method that seeks to promote health, restore energy, and balance the body-mind connection. *Qi* means the source of air, which is a vital energy for life. *Gong* means the skills and techniques that promote the natural flow and restoration of this energy. Regular qigong exercises promote better brain functioning, help blood circulation, and improve body posture (Sancier, 1994, 1996). Qigong has many procedures; each procedure is a combination of slow body movements that require body-mind concentration. This exercise works well for parents and children.

Script

Stand up, please. We are going to do a qigong exercise today. This exercise combines breathing and body movements to help you release tension and anxiety. Daily exercises will enhance blood circulation, prevent back pain, correct body posture, and prevent stomach ulcers and other digestive problems.

Stand up straight with your feet shoulder-width apart. Relax your hands. Now raise your hands toward your stomach and clasp your hands. Take a deep breath and slowly move your hands up and hold your breath. Your hands are now slowly rising in front of your mouth. Your palms are facing your mouth, and you rotate your hands so that your palms are now facing away from you. Continue to raise your hands and feel them pushing up toward the ceiling. Your arms are now fully extended, with your palms facing up and your hands still joined together. Hold your arms straight, very straight . . . and hold your breath. Now your stomach is tight and your back is straight. Your arms feel some tension, and your head is looking upright. Very good!

Now separate your hands, release your hands slowly to your sides, and exhale through your lips very slowly. Your body is exhaling all the anxiety and tension from within. Focus all your energy onto your fingertips—the energy that you would like to hold on to, the energy that you would like to use for promoting your health. As your hands are approaching your hips, you exhale all your tensions out, and you hold on to all your helpful energy. Now relax and join your hands again in front of you. Breathe normally.

When you are ready, take another deep breath, and repeat the procedure. Slowly move your hands up, up, hold it . . . hold your breath, straighten your arms, and stretch your palms to the ceiling. Now release your hands slowly to the sides, exhale slowly, and focus your energy onto your fingertips. Do this eight more times.

Slowly move your hands up, up, hold it . . . hold your breath, straighten your arms, and stretch your palms to the ceiling. Release your hands slowly to the sides, exhale slowly, and focus your energy onto your fingertips. Do this again for seven more times. [Repeat this paragraph seven more times, counting down the number of exercises remaining.]

Now you feel relaxed and your body and mind are connected. Your anxiety is gone. Relax your fingers, your arms, your toes, your legs, and your entire body.

Application

This relaxation exercise requires clients to move in slow motion. You may choose to do an imagery movement exercise with the instructions. However, guided imagery without movement may achieve only the relaxation function, not the functions for better blood circulation or body-posture restoration. Encourage clients to do this procedure or think about the slow motions of the exercise when they are experiencing stress or tension.

B25

Relaxation on the Beach

Winnie W. Y. Chan

This combination of deep breathing and guided imagery helps clients achieve a state of mental stability. It introduces a tension-free environment, and helps clients enter a deep state of relaxation. Clients learn to practice deep breathing and relaxation techniques during periods of personal stress. The exercise provides clients with an experience of well-being and inner peace as their tensions are released. Clients should be encouraged to recognize the control they have over their bodies. This exercise may also serve as an example to teach clients to explore alternative methods in dealing with life stressors. After completing this exercise, clients will find that they feel energetic as they perform their daily responsibilities.

This exercise is useful for groups of any age. In a room with enough open space, ask clients to lie on a mat or carpeted floor.

Script

Let's begin the breathing exercise. Get yourself as comfortable as possible. The first thing you need to do is take ten deep breaths. Let's try the breathing technique. Breathing in through your nose, pushing your diaphragm down, hold it and count 3, 2, 1. Now, breathing out through your mouth, count 1, 2, 3. Do it again: inhale through your nose: count 3, 2, 1; exhale through your mouth: 1, 2, 3. Now do eight more: breathe in 3, 2, 1; out 1, 2, 3; in 3, 2, 1; out 1, 2, 3. [Repeat six times.] Good!

Say to your body, "Relax." And your mind gives a silent command to your neck, relax; to your shoulders, relax; to the trunk of your body muscles, relax; to the muscles in your legs, relax; to all muscles in your body, relax. Now take a deep breath; you once again give the general command to your whole body, relax. Relax your face; relax your neck; relax your arms and hands; relax your body . . . all the muscles relax.

Now you have a good command of your body. You see yourself as an escalator slowly going down and down, feeling relaxed and calm. As you go downstairs, you count backward from ten. Count inside your mind; I'll quit counting at six, and you'll continue to count to zero. Without moving your lips, count silently with me as you are moving down from the long escalator . . . 10, going slowly . . . 9, moving down . . . 8, relaxing yourself . . . 7, taking it easy . . . 6, keep counting . . . [Silence for 5, 4, 3, 2, 1, 0.] Now you come to zero, that is the state of rest. Down to the deep state of concentration and relaxation. Relax and keep counting . . . 10, 9, 8, 7, 6, 5, 4, 3, 2, 1, 0.

As you reach relaxation, the first thing you see is a white, beautiful, private and secure beach, with beautiful flowers and the soothing sound of the ocean wave. You place a large beautiful towel on the white sand and lie down. You get as comfortable as you can. As you look up at the sky, you feel the warmth of the sun beating down on your body and penetrating the muscles. All tension seems to melt away, and it is very relaxed under the warm sun.

The sound of the wind is so pleasant. You see the sea right above the blue sky and the white clouds reflecting on the ocean; it's so peaceful. Then the ocean breeze comes blowing across the sand. And you feel the fresh, clean air kissing your cheeks. You are feeling so free and so relaxed. The healing breeze comes to massage your neck, your shoulders, your body, your fingers, your legs, and gently relax the bottoms of your feet. This healing breeze bathes every muscle and fiber. It's cleansing and healing, and you feel comfortable. As you continue to lie on the beach, you feel that all of the tensions have been blown away. And with the spirit of wind go all the anxiety, fear, and mistakes. You are totally cleansed—body, mind, and spirit. You feel light, relaxed, and happy.

As you become more relaxed, you think about all the blessings in your life. You feel very happy. At this point in your mind, you want to relax for a few minutes, for a peaceful sleep, for a sleep that rebuilds and gives you new energy and healing. Rest as long as you want to. You'll rest as you've never rested before. Now sleep, sleep with peace. When you awaken, you'll be better than you used to be. You'll feel renewed and empowered. Now come back to reality with energy and support.

Application

Music or nature sounds may facilitate the process of relaxation in this exercise. After five minutes of the exercise, ask clients to "wake up," move their eyes around, feel the relaxation, and then discuss their feelings before, during, and after the exercise. Facilitate discussions on how this exercise might be helpful in periods of stress.

If this exercise is used in a group, it may be used as an example to introduce relaxation techniques. Encourage group members to name other places they would like to go for the guided imagery and share other means of relaxation.

Realizing Your Inner Strength

Barbara J. Brandes

The purpose of this exercise is to help adolescents relax and find inner strength to resist behavior that leads to problems (e.g., substance abuse, violence, poor anger management), and to build a spiritually rich self to resist negative and explosive emotions that are counter to the behavior and life changes the adolescent has chosen to make. This exercise can be used with individuals or groups. It is important that prior to this exercise adolescents make the decision to pursue socially acceptable behavior and accept responsibility for choices.

Begin by reviewing the goals and choices that have been identified in previous therapy sessions. Remind the adolescents that, in spite of the best of intentions, at times it is difficult to keep the promises that we make to ourselves. With individuals, this script can be prerecorded with music background, and used once a day or as needed. Encourage the adolescents to use the guided imagery exercise while sitting or reclining in a comfortable room, away from noise and distraction. It is preferable for the room to be dark or dimly lit.

Script

Hello, and welcome to this tape, "Realizing Your Inner Strength." As you begin, please make certain you are in a comfortable position, either sitting or reclining. Listen to this tape in a place and at a time that you can be free from interruptions and noise.

Breathe deeply and relax completely, letting go of your troubles. Let go of any tension. Let go of anger or disappointment. Just concentrate on my voice and your own deep, slow breathing. Your eyes should be closed and your hands relaxed, not holding anything. Relax your feet. Relax your legs. Feel your abdomen and your back relax. Your arms are relaxed, and the tension in your shoulders and neck seems to melt away.

As you relax, let your mind take you to a special place—a place of your own choosing—a calm, safe place in your mind. Let the safety and comfort smooth the thoughts in your mind, allowing you to enter your inner world, a special place in your mind. Make it real with the power of your imagination. Feel the calmness as your breathing deepens. If for any reason you need more time to relax, you can stop the tape here, rewind it, and repeat the relaxation portion of this exercise.

You are now relaxed and ready to accept yourself, the world, and everyone in it. You accept the nonperfection that is human. You feel all tension leave your body. If you have any need or desire to forgive anyone, including yourself, you are ready to do so. You are aware of a sense of relief that eases your mind, opening your heart and thoughts to the potential that lies within you. You feel a calm resolve emerging from deep within—an inner strength that flows through your body. You have understanding, wisdom, and a determination to accomplish your goals. You value yourself. You are confident that you can do what you know you should do. You know what you should do, and you have the inner strength to do it. You can accomplish what you desire to accomplish. As you listen to the music, I want to imagine that you are doing what you should do and acting in harmony with your goals. You know what to do, and you do it.

Imagine you see a friend coming toward you. You know this friend will want you to do things that you choose not to do. You want to go the other way and ignore the friend, but the friend says, "Hello. Come with me." You smile but say you are busy, and you walk away. Your life is a treasure, and you are worthy of self-care. You feel good that you avoided the behavior that you no longer want. Your inner self cheers. Take a deep breath and hear in your mind, "You are wonderful! You have inner strength!" Your inner strength has guided you, and you are glad.

You continue walking. You feel yourself at peace with the world. Your inner self grows in patience and kindness. You have self-control. You act out of the abundance of your heart, with love and a type of inner peace that you do not seek to define, but accept. This peace nurtures your inner strength. You meet a new person who says things to make you angry. You want to fight or say something angry back, but you are calm and quiet. You are worthy of peace. Your inner self keeps you calm. The anger fades and you are relaxed. You take a deep breath and hear in your mind, "You are wonderful! You have inner strength!" Your inner strength has guided you. You are glad. You are at peace.

Breathe deeply. Imagine accomplishing your goals and make it real in your imagination. Let the music and your breathing nurture your inner strength as you imagine yourself doing what you need to do and staying calm when it is important to be calm. Imagine accomplishing these goals for this day, the next day, the next week, or the next year. Make it real with the power of your imagination. Let the music and your breathing nurture your inner strength as your mind lets you see yourself doing what you need to do and acting the way you choose to act so that you become the person you choose to be.

[Pause while the music continues softly for eight to ten seconds.]

You feel your inner strength, confirming that you can make the changes you need to make to accomplish your goals. See yourself successfully relying upon your inner strength to stay calm and at peace with yourself in the midst of difficulties.

[Pause while the music continues softly for five to six seconds.]

Strength and confidence flow through your body and mind. You are relaxed and calm as you picture yourself achieving your goals and becoming the person you choose to be. Listen to the music while you picture yourself acting like the person you desire to be.

[Pause while the music continues softly for ten to twelve seconds.]

Like a flower slowly unfolding, your confidence grows as you let your mind explore the feeling of successfully accomplishing your goals. You recognize the difficulties of change. You accept the challenges of your goals, and you re-affirm your decision to pursue these goals. You feel your inner wisdom and strength. Your body relaxes as you feel the strength of your convictions and learn to trust yourself to keep true to your goals. You feel a deep calm inner strength that grows stronger with each breath. [Pause.] With each breath, you nurture your inner strength, and you claim your right to achieve your goals. [Pause.] Each time you visit this special place in your mind, it will be easier to feel your inner strength and confidence. Each time you visit this special place in your mind, it will be easier to relax and depend on your inner strength. You will find it easier to treasure your life and to make decisions that support your goals. You will find it easier to trust your inner strength to guide you in your thoughts, emotions, and actions.

Any time you feel the need to visit this special place in your mind, to realize your inner strength, you have only to listen to this tape and relax, letting your inner self guide you to this special place.

Now, if you choose, you can open your eyes and listen to the music as you return to your activities of the day. If you prefer, you may drift off to sleep, relaxed and calm, aware that you have the inner strength to keep you focused on achieving your goals.

[Music continues to play.]

Application

Adolescents should be encouraged to use this exercise whenever they feel angry, tense, or discouraged by the difficulties of change. To track the effect of the guided imagery in therapy, encourage adolescents to record the effect of the exercise by journaling about the imagery. Prompt them to record how tense or relaxed they are at the beginning of the tape and at the end. These feelings could be recorded on a scale between 1 and 5, with 1 being extremely relaxed and 5 being extremely tense, anxious, or upset. Recording the effect of the exercise will help the client and you track progress, as well as provide feedback on its value.

B27

Self-Directed Relaxation

Nanette Tashnek

This experience includes a series of self-directed phrases designed to help clients quietly direct their own relaxation. This exercise is specially designed for adult groups and individuals who have physical complaints, such as tension or migraine headaches, breathing difficulties, tightness of the chest, or insomnia. It may be helpful for those who suffer from chronic tension and anxiety, who are acutely anxious in crisis situations, or who are fearful of anticipated events.

Script

Hello, welcome to a self-directed relaxation experience. At this moment, the most important thing to remember is that this is your time. Make the best use of it. You don't have to dwell on intruding thoughts. Do not think about things that have to be done, things you should have done. Put them all aside for the next few minutes. All cares and worries are put aside. Now you will try to relax your entire body, deeply and completely.

Begin by sitting on a chair with your spine rather straight. As you relax, your spine will comfortably support the weight of your body. Cross your legs or place your feet flat on the floor with your hands on your lap. Close your eyes, so you can more easily be aware of the changes that begin to take place inside your body. Allow your breathing to become regular and rhythmic. Focus on the sensations as you allow breathing to become smooth and deep. Let yourself relax as deeply as you can right now. The self-directed relaxation phrases are designed to help you relax your body, part by part. Do not attempt to force yourself to relax all at once; this will only increase the tension. During this self-directed relaxation, let yourself experience what each phrase suggests to you. During the exercise, I will read a phrase like this: my arms and hands are heavy and warm, relaxed, and warm. During the pause after each phrase, repeat the phrase mentally to yourself. Just allow yourself to feel what the phrase suggests to you. Remember, sit back and relax, deeply and completely, while remaining awake and aware.

Right now be aware of how your body feels. Start with your feet and notice how they feel right now. Be aware of the feeling in your ankles, calves, knees, thighs, hips, stomach, chest, shoulders, arms, and hands—the feelings in your neck and head. At the end of the exercise we will again go through each part of your body to observe the changes that have occurred as a result of relaxation. Let your eyes remain closed and relaxed. We will begin a journey of self-directed relaxation. As I am speaking, you are receiving messages from your body and your mind as well.

Tell yourself, "I feel quiet and easily relaxed. I am beginning to feel my relaxation deepening. My feet feel heavy and relaxed." [Pause.] If your mind begins to wander, just focus on your breathing or your heart beating. Acknowledge your thoughts, and be willing to let them go. Now continue to tell yourself, "My ankles, my knees, and my hips feel heavy, relaxed, and comfortable. My stomach and the whole central portion of my body feels relaxed and quiet. My hands, my arms, and my shoulders feel heavy, relaxed, and comfortable."

"My neck, my jaw, and my forehead feel heavy and relaxed. They feel comfortable and smooth. My whole body feels quiet, heavy, comfortable, and relaxed. I feel the weight of my whole body." Continue to allow yourself to relax even further. Let your mind be aware of the changes that are taking place inside your body. "I am more and more deeply relaxed. I feel very calm and quiet. My whole body is relaxed, and my hands are warm, relaxed and warm. My right hand is warm. Now my left hand is warm. My hands are warm. Warmth is flowing into both my hands. They are warm, warm, warm. I can feel the warmth flowing down my arms into both my hands. My hands are warm, relaxed and warm."

Continue to relax even deeper while remaining awake and aware. Continue to tell yourself, "My whole body feels heavy, warm, and relaxed. My legs and feet are heavy and warm. I can feel the warmth flowing down my legs and into my feet. My whole body is relaxed, and my feet are warm, relaxed and warm. My right and left feet are warm. My feet are warm. Warmth is flowing into both my feet. They are warm, warm, warm."

Continue to relax even deeper while remaining awake and aware. Continue to tell yourself, "My whole body feels quiet, comfortable and relaxed. My mind is passive and relaxed. I withdraw my thoughts from the surroundings, and I feel serene and still. I feel an inner sense of quietness. Deep within my mind I experience and imagine myself being relaxed, comfortable, and still. I am aware but in an easy, quiet, inward way. My mind is clear and refreshed."

Continue relaxing, more and more deeply, while remaining awake and aware. Relax freely and completely. [Pause for ten seconds with music in the background.]

In a few minutes, you'll do an exercise to reactivate yourself slowly and smoothly. Remain relaxed with your eyes closed. Without moving, be aware of how your body feels after you have allowed yourself to relax deeply. Focus your attention on your feet and on the sensations you are experiencing right now. Notice the feelings in your calves. Move on to your thighs and pelvic area, and then to your stomach. Be aware of the feelings and sensations you are feeling now in each part of your body. Continue to notice the feelings associated with deep relaxation—in your chest, arms and hands, neck and head. Notice how you feel now compared with how you felt before you started the relaxation exercise.

In the same way that you slowly relaxed yourself, it is equally important to slowly and smoothly reactivate yourself. Exhale completely now. And then take a long deep breath. As you do, feel the cool, new, fresh oxygen pouring into your body. Continue to breathe in slowly and deeply while feeling the oxygen and energy flowing into your chest, out into your hands, and down into your feet.

Continue to breathe in more deeply and more slowly, refilling your body with energy. Take a long, slow, deep breath and then exhale. Begin to wiggle your fingers and toes in order to prepare your body to become active again. Move your arms and legs. Stretch the muscles in your arms and legs. And now move the trunk of your body along with your head and neck. At your own pace, go ahead and open your eyes. Get out of the chair feeling very refreshed and very relaxed.

Application

Like any guided imagery exercise, this one helps clients restore their energy and relax in a safe environment. Encourage clients to remember deep breathing when they are facing confrontation or stressful situations. The relaxation may also be useful for those who are moderately depressed or who have difficulty controlling anger. To master this relaxation experience, prompt clients to play the prerecorded tape daily and rate their degree of relaxation. This allows them to assess their own progress.

The Tao of Guided Imagery

Patrick Leung

Taoism is an ancient Chinese philosophy that focuses on spiritual development, the concept of relativity, and an individual's relationship with nature.
Harmony and balance with nature are the most important ingredients of stress
reduction and self-development. In *I Ching,* the book of diversity and change,
storytelling is a technique used to demonstrate how people can achieve con-
sonance and balance with nature. This guided imagery exercise is adapted
from a story told by the Taoist philosopher Zhuang Zi, and it conveys the importance of self-awareness and self-respect. Use the script to help clients who
are making difficult choices, those who are going through identity crises, and
those who are experiencing stressful events. It can be used with individuals or
groups, and children with parents in a group setting.

Script

Sit in a comfortable position. Close your eyes and relax. I am going to tell you
a Taoist story. Taoists are Chinese philosophers who teach people about harmony and relationships with nature. This story begins with you sitting in a
room. This is a huge room, a very warm and comfortable room. You are relaxed. Imagine how comfortable it is and how comfortable you feel.

You meet some people there. They are your friends. You are talking with your
friends about a trip you are planning. One of your friends is a Taoist philosopher. You consult with him because he knows nature well. He says, "Just relax. Go to the mountain and you will find something of interest."

You are happy with this advice and go to the mountain. It is a giant mountain
with many trees. You notice birds singing. Two bluebirds are flying by you now.
They are beautiful. You like nature.

Next you walk toward a tree, a tree with many branches. You like this tree, but
you think it is too short. The two bluebirds fly into the tree. Their nest is built on
the branches. You now think this is a useful tree because the birds happily make
their home on its branches and leaves. You continue to walk. You are relaxed.

You see another tree in the distance. This tree is tall, but it does not have many
branches. You like this tree, but you think it is too thin. All of a sudden, the
wind blows very hard. You lean against the tree. It stands firmly and protects
you from flying away. You now think this tree is a strong tree because it protected you. You continue to walk. You are happy.

You come toward a huge tree. This tree is tall, as tall as the mountain. It has many branches, enough to provide shade for the green meadow and homes for the birds. You like this tree, but wonder why it has not been cut down to produce furniture.

You ask your Taoist friend about the differences of these trees. He answers, "Everything has its strength and potential." You think about his answer twice. "Everything has its strength and potential. Everything has its strength and potential." You don't need to make any comparisons.

Your Taoist friend tells you that the huge tree has not been cut down, because its wood is not hard enough for making furniture. If you use it to build a house, it will attract termites. If you use it for making a window frame, it will drip sap on the glass. If you use it to make a canoe, it will sink. If you use it to make a coffin, it will attract bugs. Therefore, it is allowed to continue to grow and become a beautiful, enormous tree that is appreciated by others.

Everything has its strength and potential. Everybody has his or her strength and potential, too. Something that you don't see to be useful can be the most useful thing for another person. Usefulness is a relative term because it depends on how you define it. Wow! You feel good about yourself and your surroundings. You are a useful person, you have potential to grow, and you have the strength to continue your life journey.

Now the story is ended, but you will continue to look for your destiny. You are who you are, and you learn perseverance from this experience. When you open your eyes and look around, you find yourself spiritually enriched, and you appreciate everything and every person in your surroundings. You are who you are with strength and potential!

Application

This guided imagery exercise has a Taoist spirit. Relativity is the main concept when you share the experience about decision making. It should stress the importance of appreciating one's potential. Ask the following questions as a way to process this relaxation exercise:

1. How did you feel when you saw the giant mountain, the bluebirds, the short tree, the tall but thin tree, and the huge tree?

2. Discuss the importance of balance and harmony from the experience of meeting nature.

3. How did you feel when you felt the strong wind on the giant mountain?

4. What insights did you gain from this exercise?

5. Discuss the significance of the question "Who am I?" for individuals your age.

B29

Word Association

Monit Cheung

The word-association technique has been recommended by Scott (1993) to help clients engage in free association, so that the therapist can conduct hypnoanalysis. Use this technique as an assessment tool with adolescents and adults. Explain the procedure and then read each of the chosen words slowly. In individual or group settings, each client will concentrate on each of these words and respond to them one by one. Tape this process so that clients can review their responses during treatment, if therapeutically appropriate.

Script

Close your eyes. Relax and feel comfortable. Let your mind be your guide. Relax and feel comfortable. Let your mouth speak to your mind's wisdom.

The following list is a collection of randomly selected terms and words that will assess your ability to use the unconscious mind to reflect some meaning on your current problem or situation. For example, when I say "open," you may say "close." When I say "open," you may say "well." When I say "open," you may say "door." When I say "open," you may say "open." When I say "open," you may say any word or phase that first appears in your mind, or you may say nothing at all and keep silent. I will go to the next word. When this exercise is over, I will say "Wake up" two times. You may choose to wake up at any time if you do not want to continue, or you may wake up at the end of the exercise. Let's begin now.

open	overweight	who
candy	red	escape
soft	live	abortion
bell	mouth	dominate
easy	sex	thin
father	boys	baby
life	need	guilt
fear	belief	if only
mother	my father	dance
green	anger	we
me	when	how
love	depressed	1960
blue	horrible	grandfather

sad	talent	I enjoy . . .
power	myself	feeling
girls	quick	sleeping
touch	old	wife
pain	teeth	dying
(client's name)	who	on top
feel	homosexual	year 2010
balls	must be . . .	problems
inside	time	woman
come	depressed	fighting
marriage	I became . . .	lying down
my mother	bottom	nude
pride	punishment	relax
lips	escape	ideas
dirty	desire	dry
trust	clock	husband
children	man	I hate . . .
where	big	slow
scream	party	I love . . .
home	late	wake
concerned	cheating	OK
kind	divorce	one
funeral	any name	two
water	guns	three
gentle	affection	ten
what is?	white	Wake up, wake up
black	deep	Open your eyes
grapes	lie	

Application

Word association is a psychoanalytic technique to assess clients' current situation as reflected by unconscious experiences in the past. A shorter list may be chosen for this exercise by systematically skipping some words. If clients cannot associate the word with another word or phase, stay silent for a few seconds and then go to the next word. During the counseling process, there are three important things to remember. (1) Be sure to prepare clients to return to the conscious world by using a clue such as "wake up, wake up" or counting from one to ten. (2) After you bring the client back to reality, identify and discuss repeated words or themes identified in the client's responses by asking, "Are there any specific words you can remember now?" "I notice that you used *don't know* [or other identified response] at least five times; does this term/phrase have any significant meaning to you now?" "Do you have a question about [the repeated theme]?" (3) Check with clients about their current feelings and validate these feelings with them.

B30

Your Place

Robin Doak Neyrey

This exercise is a semistructured guided imagery exercise that begins with basic body relaxation before guiding the participants to create their own place of safety and security. This exercise is effective as an opening for a group session, and as a beginning exercise for subsequent group meetings. The relaxation component allows participants to center and prepare for group work. Since a feeling of safety and support has been enhanced, group members can align their focus to work on important issues. This exercise is particularly useful as an introduction to a trauma resolution group for self-image nurturing. Soft and soothing music enhances the imagery. The Native American flute is a particularly nice accompaniment.

Script

Let's begin by sitting comfortably in your chair. It is best if you place both feet on the floor and rest your hands comfortably on your legs. Good. Begin by closing your eyes and breathing slowly in through your nose and out through your mouth. Breathe in . . . and out. In . . . and out. Breathe in relaxation and breathe out tension. Good. Keep breathing as you begin to check for tension in your body. Notice any tension in your head—the top, sides, and back of your head. Let the tension go.

Now check your face, brow, and jaw. Release all tension from your head and face. Moving down your neck, notice any tension and relax your neck. Keep breathing . . . Good! Notice any tension you may hold in your shoulders and let it go. Continuing, allow the wave of relaxation to roll over your shoulders and down your arms, through the wrists, and release all tension out the tips of your fingers. That's it . . . Good. Check the chest, stomach, and hips, releasing all tension. Notice any tightness in the thighs, knees, and lower legs. Release any tension. Your feet relax as you notice and release any tension there. You are now comfortable and relaxed. Each breath continues to bring in a deeper sense of relaxation, and each breath out dispels any remnants of tension. Your body is relaxed and comfortable.

Now in your mind's eye create for yourself a place where you are comfortable, relaxed, safe, and secure. It can be a real or imagined place. This is your special place. It is just as you want it to be. In this place you feel the warm relaxation of wholeness and tranquility. It may be a beach, a meadow, a mountaintop, or a forest . . . whatever you want it to be. Look around in your special place. Notice the colors and shapes . . . you may see towering pines, majestic mountain peaks, or endless fields of flowers. Whatever you see, notice every detail; this is your place, make it just as you would like it to be. Notice the smells, the salt of the sea, the fragrant blossoms, the earthiness of the forest floor . . . drink in every detail with your senses. Feel the textures of your special place. It may be the gentle breeze against your skin or sand under your feet or the warming sun on your skin. Notice the sounds in your comfort place—the birds singing, the waves crashing, the breeze in the trees. That's good. You can put any person or thing in your place that helps you feel safe and relaxed. It may be someone, something, even an animal or a favorite pet. All things here in your special place are there to help you feel relaxed, warm, safe, and comfortable.

Notice all the colors, shapes, textures, smells, sounds, and the very feel of your place. This special place, your place, is yours alone. In this place you are safe, secure, relaxed, and content. You feel rejuvenated by the tranquility and the beauty of your special place. This place is available to you whenever you need it. You may return here as often as you wish.

Still feeling relaxed and warmed by the wholeness of your place, you can return to the room when you are ready. Now, count down from five to ease the transition: 5 . . . You are relaxed . . . Good! . . . 4 . . . You are aware of the chair you are sitting on . . . 3 . . . You are still relaxed as you notice your senses focus back in the room . . . 2 . . . You open your eyes . . . That's it! . . . 1 . . . The comfortable feeling stays with you as you notice the other group members in the room. Excellent!

Application

This guided imagery exercise is useful as a therapeutic tool in assessment, intervention, and evaluation. Processing individuals' ability to relax and select a safety place can assess their defenses, engagement in the therapeutic alliance, and worldview. You can provide clients with a tool that is readily available for personal relaxation and self-nurturing as a therapeutic intervention that clients can exercise at will. Allowing for personal choice in the exercise is important, so that clients can enter the most beneficial setting to feel wholeness. For example, a member of a trauma resolution group may reveal the imagery of a small, dark closet in which he or she feels safe and secure. This image is contrary to the examples given in the imagery, yet it reflects this member's personal experience of safety. You can then proceed to help the client explore other choices, and discuss the richness of materials available through this imagery medium. On subsequent evaluation, clients may change their choice of a safe place and discuss its therapeutic meaning.

After the exercise, ask questions.

1. Was the relaxation exercise easy or difficult? What did you like best about the exercise?

2. Were you able to create a special/safe place? Can you tell us what makes this place special?

3. Among the five senses, which was the richest for you?

4. How has your special place changed since we started doing this exercise?

5. Have you been able to use this exercise at home? How has this been useful to you?

References

Allan, J., & Berry, P. (2002). Sand play. In C. E. Schaefer & D. Cangelosi (Eds.), *Play therapy techniques* (2nd ed., pp. 161–168). Northvale, NJ: Jason Aronson.

Bishop, D. (2005). *Derek Bishop's spiritual autobiography: Making play dough: Recipes and photos/pictures/photographs.* Retrieved January 1, 2005, from http://www.singingmountain.org/play-dough-recipes.html

Brandell, J. R. (1988). Storytelling in child psychotherapy. In C. E. Schaefer (Ed.), *Innovative interventions in child and adolescent therapy* (pp. 9–42). Oxford: John Wiley & Sons.

Buck, J. N. (1970). *The house-tree-person techniques.* Los Angeles: Western Psychological Services.

Burns, R. C., & Kaufman, S. H. (1970). *Kinetic family drawing.* New York: Brunner/Mazel.

Caruth, E. G. (1988). How you play the game: On game as play and play as game in the psychoanalytic process. *Psychoanalytic Psychology, 5*(2), 179–192.

Corey, G. (2005). *Theory and practice of counseling and psychotherapy.* Pacific Grove, CA: Brooks/Cole.

Erikson, E. (1950). *Childhood and society.* New York: Norton.

Finley, W. W., & Jones, L. C. (1992). *Handbook of clinical child psychology.* Oxford: John Wiley & Sons.

Fischetti, B. A. (2001). Use of play therapy for anger management in the school setting. In A. A. Drewes & L. J. Carey (Eds.), *School-based play therapy* (pp. 238–255). New York: John Wiley & Sons.

Freud, S. (1975). *Three essays on the theory of sexuality.* New York: Basic Books. (Original work published 1905).

Glasser, W. (1998). *Choice theory: A new psychology of personal freedom.* New York: HarperCollins.

Goldenberg, I., & Goldenberg, H. (2004). *Family therapy: An overview* (6th ed.). Pacific Grove, CA: Brooks/Cole.

Hunter, M. E. (1994). *Creative scripts for hypnotherapy.* New York: Brunner/Mazel.

Hurlock, E. B. (1972). *Child development.* New York: McGraw-Hill.

Kolhberg, L. (1981). *The philosophy of moral development: Moral stages and the idea of justice.* San Francisco: Harper & Row.

Lowry, R. J. (Ed.). (1973). *Dominance, self esteem, self actualization: Germinal papers of A. H. Maslow.* Monterey, CA: Brooks/Cole.

Mahler, M., Pine, F., & Bergman, A. (1975). *The psychological birth of the human infant: Symbiosis and individuation.* New York: Basic Books.

McDevitt, J. B., & Settlage, C. F. (1971). *Separation-individuation: Essays in honor of Margaret S. Mahler.* New York: International University Press.

Meyer, L. M. (1991). Using Gestalt therapy in the treatment of anorexia nervosa. *British Review of Bulimia & Anorexia Nervosa, 5*(1), 7–16.

Mitchell, R. R., & Friedman, H. S. (1994). *Sandplay: Past, present, and future.* New York: Routledge.

Monastra, V. J. (2005). Electroencephalographic biofeedback (neurotherapy) as a treatment for attention deficit hyperactivity disorder: Rationale and empirical foundation. *Child and Adolescent Psychiatric Clinics of North America, 14,* 55–82.

Morris, P. E., & Fritz, C. O. (2002). The improved name game: Better use of expanding retrieval practice. *Memory, 10*(4), 259–266.

Moughty, S. (2005). *The zero-to-three debate.* Retrieved March 27, 2005, from http://www.pbs.org/wgbh/pages/frontline/shows/teenbrain/science/zero.html

Murray, T. (2000). *Comparing theories of child development* (5th ed.). Belmont, CA: Wadsworth.

Newman, B. M., & Newman, P. R. (2003). *Development through life: A psychosocial approach* (8th ed.). Pacific Grove, CA: Brooks/Cole.

Olness, K., & Kohen, D. P. (1996). *Hypnosis and hypnotherapy with children* (3rd ed.). New York: Guilford Press.

Polusny, M. A., & Follette, V. M. (1996). Remembering childhood sexual abuse: A national survey of psychologists' clinical practices, beliefs, and personal experiences. *Professional Psychology: Research and Practice, 27*(1), 41–52.

Sancier, K. M. (1994). The effect of qigong on therapeutic balancing measured by electroacupuncture according to Voll (EAV). *Acupuncture and Electron-Therapeutics Research, 19,* 119–127.

Sancier, K. M. (1996). Medical applications of qigong. *Alternative Therapies, 2,* 40–45.

Satir, V. (1972). *Peoplemaking.* Palo Alto, CA: Science and Behavior Books.

Scott, J. A. (1993). *Hypnoanalysis for individual and marital psychotherapy.* New York: Gardner Press.

Shapiro, L. E. (1993). *The building blocks of self-esteem.* King of Prussia, PA: Center for Applied Psychology.

Starting Points. (1994). *Starting points: Meeting the needs of our youngest children.* New York: Carnegie Corporation.

Thompson, C. L., & Rudolph, L. B. (2004). *Counseling children.* Pacific Grove, CA: Brooks/Cole.

Webb, N. B. (1999). *Play therapy with children in crisis: A casebook for practitioners.* New York: Guilford Press.

Resources for Guided Imagery and Play Therapy

Books and Articles

Axline, V. M. (1947). *Play therapy.* New York: Ballantine.

Axline, V. M. (1949). Play therapy experiences as described by child participants. *Journal of Consulting Psychology, 14,* 53–63.

Bratton, S., & Ray, D. (2000). What research shows about play therapy. *International Journal of Play Therapy, 9*(1), 47–88.

Campbell, C. A. (1993). Play, the fabric of elementary school counseling programs. *Elementary School Guidance and Counseling, 28*(1), 10–16.

Carmichael, K. D. (1994). Sand play as elementary school strategy. *Elementary School Guidance and Counseling, 28*(4), 302–307.

Cerio, J. D. (1994). Play therapy: A brief primer for school counselors. *Journal for the Professional Counselor, 9*(2), 73–80.

Chethik, M. (2000). *Techniques of child therapy: Psychodynamic strategies* (2nd ed.). New York: Guilford Press.

Duff, S. E. (1996). A study of the effects of group family play on family relations. *International Journal of Play Therapy, 5*(2), 81–93.

Erikson, E. H. (1963). *Childhood and society* (2nd ed.). New York: Norton.

Fall, M. (1994). Physical and emotional expression: A combination approach for working with children in the small areas of a school counselor's office. *School Counselor, 42,* 73–77.

Freud, A. (1974). *Introduction to psychoanalysis: Lectures for child analysts and teachers,* 1922–1935. New York: International Universities Press.

Gil, E. (1991). *The healing power of play: Working with abused children.* New York: Guilford Press.

Gil, E. (1994). *Play in family therapy.* New York: Guilford Press.

Ginott, H. G. (1959). The theory and practice of "therapeutic intervention" in child treatment. *Journal of Consulting Psychology, 23,* 160–166.

Klein, M. (1934). The psychoanalytic play technique. *American Journal of Orthopsychiatry, 25,* 223–237.

Kottman, T. (1995). *Partners in play: An Adlerian approach to play therapy.* Alexandria, VA: American Counseling Association.

Kranz, P. L., & Lund, N. L. (1993). Axline's eight principles of play therapy revisited. *International Journal of Play Therapy, 2*(2), 53–60.

Landreth, G. L. (2000). *Innovations in play therapy.* New York: Brunner Routledge.

Landreth, G. L. (2002). *Play therapy: The art of the relationship* (2nd ed.). New York: Brunner Routledge.

Landreth, G. L., & Wright, C. S. (1997). Limit setting practices of play therapists in training and experienced play therapists. *International Journal of Play Therapy, 6,* 41–62.

Malchiodi, C. A. (Ed.). (2003). *Handbook of art therapy.* New York: Guilford Press.

Mann, D. (1996). Serious play. *Teacher's College Record, 97*(3), 446–449.

Matorin, A. I., & McNamara, J. R. (1996). Using board games in therapy with children. *International Journal of Play Therapy, 5*(2), 3–16.

McCalla, C. L. (1994). A comparison of three play therapy theories: Psychoanalytical, Jungian, and client-centered. *International Journal of Play Therapy, 3*(1), 1–10.

Moustakas, C. E. (1953). *Children in play therapy: A key to understanding normal and disturbed emotions.* New York: McGraw-Hill.

Nemiroff, M. A., & Annunziata, J. (1996). *A child's first book about play therapy.* Washington, DC: American Psychological Association.

Norton, C. C., & Norton, B. E. (2002). *Reaching children through play therapy: An experiential approach* (2nd ed.). Denver, CO: White Apple Press.

Oaklander, V. (1988). *Windows to our children* (4th ed.). Highland, NY: Gestalt Journal Press.

O'Connor, K. J. (1991). *The play therapy primer: An integration of theories and techniques.* New York: John Wiley & Sons.

Orton, G. L. (1997). *Strategies for counseling with children and their parents.* Pacific Grove, CA: Brooks/Cole.

Proulx, L. (2003). *Strengthening emotional ties through parent-child-dyad art therapy: Interventions with infants and preschoolers.* London: Jessica Kingsley.

Rogers, A. G. (1995). *A shining affliction.* New York: Viking.

Roopnarine, J. L., Johnson, J. E., & Hooper, F. H. (Eds.). (1994). *Children's play in diverse cultures.* Albany: State University of New York Press.

Schaefer, C. E. (Ed). (2002). *Play therapy with adults.* Hoboken, NJ: John Wiley & Sons.

Tanner, Z., & Mathis, R. D. (1995). A child-centered typology for training novice play therapists. *International Journal of Play Therapy, 4*(2), 1–13.

Webb, W. (1992). Empowering at-risk children. *Elementary School Guidance and Counseling, 27,* 96–103.

Van de Putte, S. J. (1995). A paradigm for working with child abuse survivors of sexual abuse who exhibit sexualized behaviors during play therapy. *International Journal of Play Therapy, 4*(1), 27–49.

Van Fleet, R. (2000). Understanding and overcoming parent resistance to play therapy. *International Journal of Play Therapy, 9*(1), 35–46.

Internet Resources: Organizations

American Association for the Study of Mental Imagery
http://www.uml.edu/dept/psychology/aasmi/

Association for Music and Imagery
http://www.bonnymethod.com/ami/

Association for Play Therapy
http://www.a4pt.org/

British Association of Play Therapists
http://www.bapt.info/

Canadian Association for Child and Play Therapy
http://www.cacpt.com/

International Expressive Arts Therapy Association
http://www.ieata.org/index.html

International Imagery Association
http://www.imagery-iia.com/

International Society for Child and Play Therapy
http://www.playtherapy.org/

National Expressive Therapy Association
http://www.expressivetherapy.com/index_other.html

Sandplay Therapists of America
http://www.sandplay.org/index.htm

Internet Resources: Professional Training

Academy for Guided Imagery
http://www.academyforguidedimagery.com/faqs.php

Center for Play Therapy, University of North Texas
http://www.coe.unt.edu/cpt/

Chesapeake Beach Professional Seminars
http://www.cbpseminars.com/

Family and Play Therapy Center
http://www.fptcenter.com/

Imagery Training Institute
http://imagery-training-institute.com/

Integrative Imagery Training for Health Care Professionals
http://www.integrativeimagery.com/index.htm

Kid Power
http://www.playtherapycentral.com/

The Play Therapy Training Institute
http://www.ptti.org/

The Theraplay Institute
http://www.theraplay.org/

Internet Resources: Professional Materials

Anna's Toy Depot
http://www.annastoydepot.com/

Bright Spots Games
http://www.brightspotsgames.com/

Childswork/Childsplay
http://www.childswork.com/

ChildTherapyToys.com
http://www.childtherapytoys.com/

Dye-namic Movement Products
http://www.dyenamicmovement.com/

ePlayTherapy.com
http://www.eplaytherapy.com/

Family Enhancement and Play Therapy Center
http://www.play-therapy.com/

Guided Imagery, Inc.
http://www.guidedimageryinc.com/

Health Journeys
http://www.healthjourneys.com/

Inner Vision Studio, Inc.
http://www.innervisionstudioinc.com/

Peaceful Awareness
http://peacefulawareness.com/index.htm

Serenity Music
http://www.serenitymusic.com/

Toys of the Trade
http://www.toysofthetrade.com/shopping/agora.cgi

About the Author and Contributors

Monit Cheung, MA, MSW, PhD, LCSW, is professor and chair of the children and families concentration at the University of Houston Graduate College of Social Work in Houston, Texas. She specializes in child sexual abuse counseling, play therapy, and family therapy. She has 30 years of practice, teaching, research, and administrative experience in the fields of children's mental health, children's protective services, and psychotherapy practice. Cheung has written books on child psychology, child development, cultural development, and parenting techniques for Chinese parents. She currently serves as board member and chair of advocacy committee at the Catholic Charities in Houston and board member and life member of End Child Sexual Abuse Foundation in Hong Kong.

Mark F. Akerlund, LCSW, is the Houston and Dallas/Fort Worth coordinator for Social Work prn, a professional social work company that provides temporary staffing services for social workers. He also has a private practice and provides supervision, consulting, and psychotherapy services to various agencies in the Houston area.

Yolanda Alvarado, LMSW, is director of education at Planned Parenthood of Houston and Southeast Texas. She has eighteen years of experience as an instructor/trainer and in program implementation in the fields of human sexuality, family planning, reproductive health, and teenage pregnancy.

Kay Anderson, BS, has been with Child Advocates, Inc., in Houston, Texas, since 1989. She is the program manager and advocacy coordinator, and helps train and supervise volunteers who are appointed as guardians *ad litem* for abused and neglected children in the custody of the Texas Department of Family and Protective Services.

Kelli L. Beveridge, MSW, has been working for the State of Texas, including Children's Protective Services, since 1999. She is a clinical and political advocate for children traumatized by sexual abuse.

Barbara J. Brandes, MPA, LMSW, ASOTP, is a therapist at ADAPT Counseling, working with sexual abuse survivors and families. She is also an expert in counseling adolescents with disciplinary, sexual, and behavior problems.

Winnie W. Y. Chan, MSW, LMSW, is social work officer, Planning and Coordinating Team, at the Social Welfare Department, Hong Kong. Her clinical interest is in assessing family dynamics and enhancing family competence.

Renata Domatti, LMSW, CMM, is case manager at Cornerstone Hospital of Central Texas. She guides patients through the healing process.

Demori Currid Driver, BA, is research associate at the University of Houston Graduate College of Social Work and a public health student at the University of Texas Health Science Center at Houston. She is a former elementary school teacher, works with children and their families, and has enthusiastically used play therapy in her practice.

Kristin Geiss-Curran is an MSW alumnus at the University of Houston Graduate School of Social Work. She has worked to help children and families involved in adoption, crisis pregnancy, and substance abuse.

Molly Grimmer, MSW, LMSW, is a school social worker. She has been a social worker since 1992, and has worked in child welfare settings with sexually abused children and their families.

Colleen Knox, LCSW, has worked with adolescents and their families in a residential treatment center and in foster homes. In addition, she has experience counseling women with eating disorders, living with violent partners, and making major life transitions.

Patrick Leung, PhD, MSW, MA, BSSW, is associate professor and former doctoral program director at the University of Houston Graduate College of Social Work, where he teaches research, statistics, program evaluation, and policy analysis. He has had extensive experience in child welfare research and program evaluations.

Sandra A. Lopez, LCSW, ACSW, is clinical associate professor at the University of Houston Graduate College of Social Work. She also is a diplomat in clinical social work in clinical practice in the Houston area, and has developed expertise in working with grieving children and their families.

Kit-Ying Anny Ma, LMSW, social worker in Optional Practical Training, is interested in multicultural practice, family preservation, and domestic violence issues. She has provided social services to children and families in schools, family service centers, and transitional living centers in Hong Kong and the United States.

Othea G. McCoy-Clinton, LMSW, is therapist for the Harris County Juvenile Probation Department. She has been working in the social services field for over 20 years, as an advocate for children and youth institutionalized within the judicial system, and for the care and well-being of the elderly.

Susan E. McCullough, LCSW, Certified Personal Life Coach, is a psychotherapist in private practice. She has experience as a mental health professional in both nursing homes and schools.

Tracy A. Middleton, MEd, is a former educator and has provided counseling services to children and adolescents while working at a county mental health facility. She is currently a law student with an interest in juvenile law.

Ed Muldrow, PhD, LCSW, is family therapist for the Department of Psychiatry at Mainland Medical Center, and works extensively with the Children Cope with Divorce Program in Houston and Galveston. He is a faculty member in the School of Human Services at University of Phoenix and Capella University.

Laila Amir Narsi, LCSW, is a psychotherapist in private practice in the greater Houston area. Her specialties include multicultural studies, women's issues, and anxiety and stress management.

Robin Doak Neyrey, LMSW, is social worker at Tomball Regional Hospital in both the physical rehabilitation and mental health units.

Wing-Sai Dion Or, MSW, is assistant to the director, International Affairs and Development, Mayor's Office, City of Houston. She has worked with youth at risk, school dropouts, drug addicts, and juvenile offenders.

Patricia R. Palmer, MA, LCSW, is a social worker and psychotherapist in practice in Houston, Texas. She is interested in mindfulness and meditation as sources of healing, empowerment, and peace.

Sharon Clark Peska, LGSW, is a hospice social worker at Jewish Social Service Agency in Rockville, Maryland. She provides emotional support for people who are near the end of their life, and for their families.

Heather Alden Pope, LGSW, is school social worker at St. Paul Public Schools in Minnesota. She is also an on-call worker in a children's hospital. She is a former teacher and lifelong advocate for equality in education.

Jolene L. Pothier, MEd, is a licensed professional counselor, and is interested in working with adolescents.

Lori Swan Provence, LMSW, is a case manager with the Buckner Children and Family Services Foster Care Program.

Alyssa I. Sanders, MA, MSW, is special assistant to the president and CEO of Neighborhood Centers, Inc. She is a political social worker, and is interested in women's rights.

Laura G. Saunders, LMSW, LCDC, has been a social worker with children and families since 1982. She is family group decision-making program director, Child Protective Services, Department of Family and Protective Services in Houston, Texas. She also supervises the Family Group Conferencing Specialists and Kinship Caregiver Specialists, who work with relatives and fictive kin who are caring for children in protective custody.

Nanette Tashnek, LCSW, specializes in alternative therapies. She is a practitioner of Radix body-oriented personal growth work, and a trainer in eidetic image therapy.

Beth Tauber, MSW, is developing her social work practice through the Children's Crisis Care Center. She conducts developmental assessments on abused and neglected children six years old and younger.

Michele Ostrowski Taylor, LMSW, has worked with children and adolescents in a variety of therapeutic settings, including foster care, residential treatment, therapeutic horseback riding, and individual and family counseling.

Amy L. Thompson, LMSW, is a caseworker in a sexual abuse unit of Children's Protective Services. She is also the director of a volunteer organization that provides peer support for gay/lesbian youth.

Laura Tolle, LCSW, is a consultant for at-risk youth in Houston, Texas. She has trained staff in child behavior management.

Mary Elisia Wu graduated from Trinity University with a BS in international business and a minor in Chinese. She is attending Loyola Marymount University, where she is pursuing a master of arts in elementary education.

Index of Exercises